IBS

All New Content

by Kristina Campbell, MSc;
Maitreyi Raman, MD, FRCPC; and
Natasha Haskey, RD, PhD

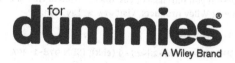

A Wiley Brand

IBS For Dummies®

Published by: **John Wiley & Sons, Inc.**, 111 River Street, Hoboken, NJ 07030-5774, www.wiley.com

For general information on our other products and services, please contact our Customer Care Department within the U.S. at 877-762-2974, outside the U.S. at 317-572-3993, or fax 317-572-4002. For technical support, please visit https://hub.wiley.com/community/support/dummies.

Wiley publishes in a variety of print and electronic formats and by print-on-demand. Some material included with standard print versions of this book may not be included in e-books or in print-on-demand. If this book refers to media that is not included in the version you purchased, you may download this material at http://booksupport.wiley.com. For more information about Wiley products, visit www.wiley.com.

Library of Congress Control Number: 2025933257

ISBN 978-1-394-28945-5 (pbk); ISBN 978-1-394-28947-9 (ebk); ISBN 978-1-394-28946-2 (ebk)

SKY10099734_031025

Contents at a Glance

Recipes at a Glance

Desserts

Vegetarian

Table of Contents

Introduction

In the Western world, the separateness of the body and the brain is constantly reinforced: Schoolchildren are taught about digestive tract anatomy and physiology separately from that of the brain. Different medical specialties exist for the gut (gastroenterology) and the brain (psychiatry). The typical medicines that treat brain-related conditions such as depression are designed to target receptors in the brain, not in the rest of the body. For better or for worse, many people operate on the assumption that the body (including the digestive tract) and the brain exist in completely different boxes.

Yet, the oneness of body, mind, and spirit has been a fundamental tenet of some Eastern belief systems for thousands of years. In India, for example, the practice of yoga emerged from the knowledge that body, mind, and spirit are interconnected. Ayurveda, Chinese traditional medicine, and other ancient practices have found success in supporting health by treating the body and the brain as inseparable.

The existence of irritable bowel syndrome (IBS) reinforces the impossibility of truly separating the body from the brain. The scientists who study the complex ways in which the gut and the brain relate to each other in this condition are hard-pressed to say where brain biology stops and body biology begins, because they are, in fact, intertwined. In IBS, the body and the brain are constantly communicating in multiple, overlapping ways, including through nerve activation, immune cells, and chemical messengers.

The Western medical community's understanding of IBS has come a long way during the past four decades. After a group of doctors and researchers in the 1980s demanded better answers and consensus, IBS went from a disorder that was seen as psychological in origin and accompanied by serious stigma, to a legitimate gut-brain problem that is known to affect quality of life for more than one in ten people worldwide. The medical status of IBS in the current era is ultimately a success story of doctors listening to their patients and — despite a lack of data that would lead them in one direction or another — deciding to unite around a clinical path forward.

What doctors and scientists know about IBS has changed and continues to change. This book brings together the latest understandings of IBS and helps reintegrate ideas about the digestive system and the brain. The book is also packed with practical, evidence-based actions to help you get a handle on your IBS. So, if you have IBS or suspect you have IBS, you've come to the right place.

Even if you're not used to discussing gut health symptoms and IBS with anyone in real life, we've got your back. This book describes IBS in a clear and straightforward manner, giving you the words to understand and talk about what's happening with your symptoms. This is a judgment-free space to explore the entire picture of your wellness and how it may be affected by your experiences with IBS.

The best thing you can do when you have IBS is to arm yourself with more knowledge. And the book you have in your hands is a big part of that. With credible information at your fingertips, you'll better understand your symptoms and what's behind them so you can embrace your diagnosis with open arms and make progress in your wellness. We're honored that you've come along on this journey.

About This Book

In the past if you were looking through the bookstore shelves for a resource on IBS, you'd likely have found books that focused on the digestive aspects of IBS and had only brief coverage of brain-related factors such as stress.

IBS For Dummies is a unique resource that offers you the latest thinking about IBS, with an emphasis on how you can target both your gut and your brain to feel better. This book brings together a wealth of information from scientific studies, as well as knowledge from Maitreyi and Natasha's clinical experience, written by Kristina in a fun and readable tone, to create an indispensable resource for helping you get a handle on your IBS. In classic *For Dummies* style, there's no pressure to read the whole book from start to finish. Leave the book somewhere in your living space (just saying, beside the toilet isn't the worst idea) and flip to any page to pick up some tips when you have a few minutes.

In the Recipes in This Book and Recipes in This Chapter lists, you'll see a tomato icon (🍅) next to some recipe titles. This icon indicates that the recipe is vegetarian.

Finally, within this book, you may note that some web addresses break across two lines of text. If you're reading this book in print and you want to visit one of these web pages, simply key in the web address exactly as it's noted in the text, pretending as though the line break doesn't exist. If you're reading this as an e-book, you've got it easy — just click the web address to be taken directly to the web page.

Foolish Assumptions

When writing this book, the authors make the following assumptions about you:

» You're experiencing IBS-like symptoms and you may or may not have received an official diagnosis of IBS. We cover why getting a medical diagnosis is a critical step toward wellness and how you can go about it.

» You'd prefer to be free of your symptoms, so you're looking for treatments that are supported by evidence showing they're safe and effective.

» You're open to taking charge of your diet to improve IBS symptoms. You want to implement the research showing that diet can be effective for managing symptoms, and you also want to eat tasty, colorful meals.

Icons Used in This Book

Throughout this book you'll see the following icons to draw your attention to certain paragraphs:

WARNING

When you see the Warning icon, pay attention — it tells you something that could help prevent problems when you're dealing with IBS.

TIP

The Tip icon highlights a practical thing you can do to improve your wellness or deal with IBS.

TECHNICAL STUFF

The Technical Stuff icon flags detailed (nonessential) information about IBS for anyone who wants to dig deeper into the science. If you're short on time, you can skip these paragraphs without missing anything crucial to your understanding of the subject at hand.

REMEMBER

The Remember icon marks an important point to pay attention to if you're skimming through the book and just want to catch the highlights.

Beyond the Book

In addition to the information in this book, you get access to even more help and information online at Dummies.com. Check out this book's Cheat Sheet for a quick summary of IBS management and the dietary approaches that may bring you relief. Just go to www.dummies.com and type **IBS For Dummies Cheat Sheet** in the Search box.

Where to Go from Here

The structure of this book allows you to start reading on any page and pick up useful information without a lot of background knowledge. Starting with Chapter 2 will give you a good grounding in the definition of IBS and how to describe the symptoms. If you want to get more technical and understand the mechanisms of how your gut and your brain communicate with each other, you can jump in and start reading at Chapter 4.

If you don't yet have an IBS diagnosis, check out Chapter 5, which walks you through why diagnosis is crucial and what to expect when you seek help from a medical professional.

If you're not sure where to begin, flip through the table of contents or the index and find a topic that calls to you. And don't forget, any time you come across a word that's unfamiliar to you, check for it in the glossary.

Finally, if you want to go beyond IBS symptoms and learn about general gut health, check out Kristina's book *Gut Health For Dummies* (John Wiley & Sons) for guidelines and lifestyle tips that address general gut health at all ages. If you want to share feedback on this book with the authors, please contact Kristina through her website: www.bykriscampbell.com.

We're thrilled you have this book in your possession, and we hope you come away with a deeper understanding of IBS and a clear idea of ways to move forward.

1

Becoming Familiar with IBS

Find the definition of IBS and what symptoms can occur.

Figure out what puts you at risk for IBS and what scientists know about the underlying causes.

Get a handle on how the gut-brain axis works and how it's disrupted in IBS.

Chapter **1**

A Road Map to Success with IBS

Under normal circumstances, the brain and the digestive tract (or gut) are good buddies. They send messages back and forth all day long — sharing the minutiae of what you're eating and your emotional state, giving thumbs-up emojis when everything's going well and warning each other when they sense trouble.

But in someone with irritable bowel syndrome (IBS), the communication between the gut and the brain is much more chaotic. The gut may send a very routine message that a sip of coffee is incoming, and the brain responds with an all-out emergency alarm, sending signals to speed up the muscle contractions in the gut and prepare for a bowel movement. Or the gut may sense a small, normal bubble of air and kick up the drama, telling the brain to activate its pain centers. In fact, different sensations in the gut all day long may be interpreted as signals to activate pain-sensitive regions of the brain.

IBS (not to be confused with inflammatory bowel disease, or IBD) is a disorder of gut-brain interaction (DGBI), which involves disruption in the normal two-way communication that should proceed seamlessly between the gut and the brain.

This chapter is an overview of what IBS is, why it's important to receive a diagnosis, and how to manage IBS using a holistic approach that encompasses your diet and other aspects of your lifestyle.

Comprehending IBS

Over the past 200 years, doctors and scientists have gradually come to understand more about the pattern of symptoms that characterizes IBS and how the symptoms arise. IBS was previously known as a functional disorder (with no known physical cause), but now it's better understood as a DGBI.

Discovering what defines IBS

IBS is best perceived as a cluster of digestive symptoms that indicate faulty gut-brain communication. Individuals with IBS may have very different underlying factors contributing to these symptoms.

No physical damage to the digestive tract is observed in IBS. As outlined in Chapter 2, the defining features of IBS are as follows:

>> Abdominal pain that's related to bowel movements.

>> Abnormal bowel movements, either more or less often than normal for you, or with a different appearance than usual; the bowel movements may be loose and watery or hard and lumpy.

Outside of these core symptoms, people with IBS often experience other gastrointestinal (GI) symptoms such as bloating, distension, intestinal gas, and burping.

Although IBS is not a life-threatening condition, it can have an outsize effect on your quality of life. Proper diagnosis is essential, and treatment should be approached with seriousness and determination.

Pinpointing who tends to get IBS and why

In the United States, researchers estimate that around 6 percent of adults have a diagnosis of IBS and about 15 percent live with IBS-like symptoms. Rates of IBS are different in various countries around the world and tend to change over time.

Chapter 3 covers various risk factors that increase someone's chance of developing IBS.

Although the root cause of IBS is complex, the following biological changes are sometimes seen (inconsistently) in people with IBS:

>> **Abnormal GI motility:** Motility is how quickly food and fluids move through the digestive tract with the help of gut muscles. Motility disruptions can result in diarrhea (if too fast) or constipation (if too slow).

>> **Increased sensitivity to pain or discomfort in the digestive tract:** In people with IBS, scientists have found increased sensitivity to pain, and/or activation of the brain's pain centers in response to normal, non-painful gut stimuli.

>> **A more permeable gut barrier:** The gut barrier usually seals off the digestive tract from the rest of the body while retaining spaces between cells that can open up to let in essential nutrients and water. Some people with IBS have a more permeable (or leaky) gut barrier, leading to symptoms that include abdominal pain.

>> *Dysregulation* **(abnormal cell activity) of the immune system:** Even though IBS is not associated with abnormal clinical measures of inflammation, some people with IBS have different patterns of immune cell activation than people without IBS.

>> **Pelvic floor dysfunction:** Some cases of IBS are associated with pelvic floor muscles not working properly, contributing to diarrhea or constipation.

>> **Difficulty digesting or absorbing some carbohydrates:** Some people with IBS show disrupted chemistry in the small intestine, which causes certain carbohydrates to be poorly absorbed and leads to the production of gases and water to result in diarrhea. Others may lack the enzymes (chemicals) to break down specific carbohydrates such as the lactose in dairy products, causing digestive symptoms.

>> **Changes in the community of gut microbes:** Studies have found differences in the types and amounts of microorganisms in the digestive tracts of people with IBS, compared with healthy people. These microorganisms help regulate the immune system and other body functions such as motility, so their disruption may cause gut symptoms.

Understanding how the gut-brain axis works

IBS is characterized by a breakdown in the functioning of the gut-brain axis, the two-way communication channel that extends between the digestive tract and the brain. Chapter 4 delves into the components of the gut-brain axis and how they work together.

The main parts of your digestive tract, from top to bottom, are:

>> Oral cavity (mouth)

>> Esophagus

>> Stomach

>> Small intestine

>> Large intestine

Other organs, such as the liver and pancreas, also make important contributions to digestion. However, the digestive tract itself maintains a stable environment by managing two main functions: digestion and *absorption* (letting things in) along with *defense* (keeping things out). It manages these functions with the help of several other important but lesser-known systems: the gut's own nervous system, called the *enteric nervous system* (ENS); gut microorganisms; the immune system; and the enteroendocrine system.

The main channels of two-way communication between the gut and the brain are:

>> **Nerve activation:** ENS neurons interact with the *vagus nerve,* which is the main superhighway for gut-brain messages.

>> **Immune signals:** Immune cells from the gut can release signals that reach the brain.

>> **Hormone and other molecule signals:** Various hormones and other molecules (called *metabolites*) produced in the gut can activate ENS neurons and convey messages to the brain. These molecules may also circulate in the blood and reach targets in the brain.

Some of these modes of communication are disrupted in IBS.

Navigating a Diagnosis of IBS

If you have IBS-like symptoms, seeking an official IBS diagnosis is important because it allows you to rule out closely related conditions that require very different treatments. Chapters 5 and 6 correct the record on the misunderstandings around IBS diagnosis.

Getting diagnosed

Diagnosis by a medical professional is a critical first step in taking charge of your IBS. Other conditions — such as celiac disease, colorectal cancer, endometriosis, IBD, small intestinal bacterial overgrowth, and thyroid disorders — may look similar to IBS but require very different treatments, so they should be ruled out before proceeding. Chapter 5 walks through the typical process of IBS diagnosis.

No single test positively confirms that you have IBS, so diagnosis involves two phases:

» Confirming symptoms that fit the IBS pattern

» Ruling out other conditions that may account for the symptoms

The diagnosis may be confirmed only after the symptoms occur for six months or more.

TIP

When seeking a diagnosis, keeping a written log is the best way to track your symptoms in the days and weeks before your doctor's appointment.

A medical history is usually the first step in IBS diagnosis. Then, after your doctor conducts a physical examination, some or all of the following tests may be carried out:

» Cross-sectional imaging (such as an abdominal ultrasound)

» Blood tests

» Stool tests

» Endoscopic evaluations

After this information is collected, the doctor puts the pieces together and determines whether an IBS diagnosis is appropriate. During the process of diagnosis, be cautious about implementing dietary changes prematurely because they can negatively affect some test results.

Knowing what to expect after diagnosis

Receiving a diagnosis of IBS can leave you wondering "What's next?" You may feel relieved to know the name of your condition, overwhelmed by the thought of starting to change your lifestyle, and many other emotions. As Chapter 6 explains, after diagnosis you begin a personal emotional journey as you embrace a new way of understanding your health. During this journey, you can deliberately adjust your mindset to set you up for positive action and give you the best chance of success.

Some simple actions may help you accept the diagnosis and embrace your feelings about it, helping you move forward positively and proactively:

>> Naming your emotions

>> Gaining more (science-backed) information about IBS

>> Committing to care for yourself

TIP

Every person with IBS deserves care and support, and after you're diagnosed you may find it helpful to create a list of people who can support you in various ways throughout your IBS journey. Typically this list may include:

>> Primary care provider

>> Specialist physicians

>> Registered dietitian

>> Other medical professionals

>> Alternative healthcare providers

>> Household members

>> Family members or friends

>> Other people with IBS

Approaching IBS Treatment

The state-of-the-art approach to IBS treatment involves adjusting your diet and other aspects of your lifestyle to normalize gut-brain communication. Unfortunately, no magic pill exists that will resolve all IBS symptoms. But viewed in a positive way, this lifestyle approach to treating IBS may mean you'll end up with your symptoms more under control while being healthier and more resilient overall. And as the science continues to progress, some treatment options may be refined or added to the list.

Changing your diet

Changing what and how you eat is a very effective lifestyle solution to gain control over your IBS symptoms, and Chapter 7 goes over the basics of dietary change for IBS management.

Before you significantly change the foods you eat, a first step for IBS management is to consider some simple strategies around how you eat:

>> Implementing regular mealtimes

>> Avoiding overeating and undereating

>> Eating mindfully, free of distractions

Then you may decide to implement some basic dietary changes, advisable for many people with IBS, that probably won't interfere with your overall nutritional intake:

>> Staying hydrated by drinking enough water

>> Reducing your intake of alcohol, caffeine, and carbonated drinks

>> Avoiding artificial sweeteners and ultra-processed foods that contain many additives

>> Limiting fatty and fried foods

If you implement these basic changes and your symptoms still persist, you may want to consider making a bigger change in your overall dietary pattern.

Your most important tool when you make dietary changes is a food diary, which is a list of all the foods you consume over a certain time period. A food diary helps you track your progress and decide if your dietary change is worthwhile.

Choosing a specific diet for IBS management

Dietary change in IBS has the potential to reduce the burden of gut-irritating foods in your digestive tract, enabling gut-brain communication to proceed more smoothly. However, people with IBS should take care not to overly restrict their diet because they may put themselves at risk for a nutritional deficiency.

According to current research, the most effective diet for improving IBS symptoms is called low-FODMAP (*FODMAP* stands for *fermentable oligosaccharides, disaccharides, monosaccharides, and polyols*). However, several other diets are easier to implement and may give you almost as much relief from symptoms. Chapter 8 goes over the specific diets that are shown to reduce IBS symptoms, but here's a quick overview:

>> **NICE diet:** Relatively easy to implement, this diet reduces symptoms almost as much as a low-FODMAP diet. This diet entails restricting bothersome items such as caffeine and high-fiber foods, and eating mindfully with small, regular meals.

>> **Low-FODMAP diet:** This fairly restrictive diet is highly effective for reducing IBS symptoms and involves three separate phases: restriction, reintroduction, and personalization. However, the restricted foods are not intuitive, so it takes extra effort and guidance to make sure you're adhering to it.

>> **FODMAP gentle diet:** This is a toned-down version of a full low-FODMAP diet. FODMAP gentle involves removing key high-FODMAP foods from the diet and is relatively easy to implement on your own.

>> **Gluten-free diet:** This diet eliminates only gluten, so it's easier to grasp and implement than the low-FODMAP diet. Wheat (a major source of FODMAPs in most people's diets) is not allowed.

>> **Mediterranean diet:** This well-rounded diet is focused on fruits, vegetables, whole grains, nuts, seeds, olive oil, and fatty fish, which can help maintain the health of the gut. It's a proven diet for supporting long-term health, although it may only reduce IBS symptoms to a modest degree.

Chapter 17 is packed with practical tips to help you succeed at the challenging task of changing your diet. For delicious snack and meal options that are low-FODMAP, Chapters 18 through 21 feature a collection of recipes you can incorporate into your dietary planning.

Navigating medications

Several medications are available for treating IBS, and many people with IBS include a medication as part of their comprehensive IBS management plan to stabilize their symptoms over the long term. Some medications target IBS in general, while others are specific to IBS-C or IBS-D. Chapter 9 breaks down the different types of medications (and supplements) that are shown to reduce symptoms.

REMEMBER

When considering medications for helping you manage your IBS, remember that no IBS medication works for everyone and most of the available medications have a modest effect. Trial and error may be necessary to find the medication that works best for you.

Some of the nonprescription products shown to improve IBS symptoms include:

>> Antidiarrheals

>> Bulking agents

>> Peppermint oil

>> Specific probiotics

Categories of prescription medications demonstrated to improve IBS symptoms are:

>> Antibiotics

>> Antidiarrheals

>> Antispasmodics

>> Neuromodulators

>> Promotility agents

>> Secretagogues

See Chapter 9 for more information about these medications.

Exploring emerging treatments

Some treatments (certain herbal supplements, for example) don't currently have a lot of scientific evidence showing they work, so they're considered emerging treatments for IBS. As Chapter 10 discusses, some of these treatments seem compelling because they're recommended to you through word of mouth or supported by testimonials in marketing materials or on social media. You may decide to try one or more of these treatments (as long as they're safe), but be sure to discuss them beforehand with your doctor.

Seeking mind-body treatments

With IBS symptoms often being sensitive to stress and mood, a missing piece of the treatment puzzle for many people with IBS is an intervention that targets the brain.

Mind-body interventions are brain retraining techniques that help improve neural pathways to normalize your body's function. These treatments target the two-way messages that travel through the gut-brain axis, creating a way to calm both the brain and body simultaneously. They work by restoring the balance between *sympathetic* (fight-or-flight) and *parasympathetic* (rest-and-digest) nervous system functions and normalizing pain processing in the brain.

REMEMBER

An overall aim for those with IBS can be to develop mindfulness (intentionally making yourself focus on the present moment while accepting all your thoughts and emotions), which leads to improvements in the severity of IBS symptoms, a better quality of life, and less pronounced anxiety.

The following mind-body interventions are scientifically demonstrated to help you reduce IBS symptoms:

>> Clinical hypnosis or gut-directed hypnotherapy

>> Cognitive behavioral therapy (unlearning the negative thoughts and behaviors around your gut symptoms and stress)

>> Breathing exercises

>> Meditation

>> Mindfulness-based stress reduction

>> Yoga

Adjusting your lifestyle

Your lifestyle is your overall collection of habits and behaviors together with your living conditions. It's the most significant factor in helping you manage your IBS. If you've already implemented both diet and mind-body treatments, Chapter 12 delves into how to change other aspects of your lifestyle for IBS management.

Besides diet and mind-body interventions, the lifestyle factors most likely to have an impact on your IBS symptoms are:

>> Daily moderate-intensity physical activity/exercise

>> Proper sleep (seven to nine hours per night)

>> Staying healthy by avoiding infections

Adjusting your toilet position and technique can also make a difference for some people with IBS. Plus, you may decide to incorporate professional services such as massage into your lifestyle if they're accessible to you.

Maximizing your quality of life

Beyond all the IBS treatment strategies described in this book, which work synergistically to improve symptoms, you can employ other strategies to help improve your quality of life overall as you live with IBS. The number-one factor for improving your quality of life with IBS is maintaining your social contact and supports. Plus, because IBS is so prevalent across the population, many new tools and supports have emerged specifically for IBS management. Chapter 13 has a wealth of tools, services, tips, and tricks to make your life easier; you can find out how to navigate different situations at home, at work, at school, in public places, in others' homes, while eating out, while traveling, or during dating and intimacy. After you read through Chapter 13, you can also look to Chapter 22 for ten must-have items for your day-to-day survival with IBS.

Managing IBS in Special Cases

Certain special cases may require adjustments to how IBS is managed:

>> **IBS in childhood:** Anywhere between 3 percent and 25 percent of children have IBS-like symptoms, with only a subset of them receiving an IBS diagnosis. Rest assured, most children with IBS grow and develop in an normal way. The diagnosis and treatment of IBS in children is largely the same as it is in adults, but Chapter 14 outlines a few key considerations for kids. Clear communication between the child, parent/caregiver, and doctor is essential for proper management of IBS. For the best outcomes, manage IBS symptoms by adjusting the child's diet, environment, and other lifestyle factors such as physical activity. The foundational principles of diet for children with IBS are to eat calmly and mindfully, establish good nutrition and hydration, and avoid any specific foods that trigger symptoms.

>> **IBS during pregnancy:** People with IBS may find that, during pregnancy, their symptoms stay the same, get worse, or improve. IBS doesn't harm the baby or cause negative outcomes. Chapter 15 covers how to plan for pregnancy when you have IBS, as well as how to manage during pregnancy and in the postpartum period. Before pregnancy, your goal should be to have your IBS symptoms as well controlled as possible. During pregnancy, proper nutrition and hydration are essential, even if you have to work around certain foods that

trigger symptoms. Keeping your body and mind relaxed is important for good pregnancy outcomes, as well as for reducing IBS symptoms. Check with a doctor or pharmacist before starting to take any medications or supplements for IBS during pregnancy.

>> **IBS in athletes:** High levels of athletic performance put stress on the body and frequently cause GI symptoms in normal, healthy athletes, making bowel urgency a common problem. However, athletes with IBS may face additional challenges. But as Chapter 16 explains, IBS doesn't have to stand in the way of high athletic performance. If you experience more gut symptoms as you train harder, you may make adaptations such as bathroom stops along your route or looser clothing while you train. Athletes with IBS also have to balance their high requirement for energy intake with avoidance of gut-irritating foods. Before competitions, avoid your personal triggers as well as common gut-disrupting foods. You may also decide to experiment with the timing of your meals to minimize gut symptoms as you train and compete.

Chapter **2**

Demystifying IBS

I n a book or movie, an irritable character is easy to spot. They react with angry annoyance to seemingly random things — bright sunlight, a few drops of spilled coffee, the sound of someone chewing. Such a character is abnormally sensitive to experiences that most other people would barely notice.

If you have irritable bowel syndrome (IBS), your digestive tract may share traits with this classic character type. Your digestive tract may be extra-sensitive, surprising you with symptoms such as pain and bloating when you did nothing extraordinary to provoke it. Maybe you wake up in the morning with your bowel saying, "I can't believe you thought it was a good idea to eat watermelon last night" or "You know you're the one who's going to make or break that important work project, right?" Everyday activities and milestones may prove bothersome to your bowel, giving you no choice but to spend extra effort caring for it and keeping the peace.

This chapter dives into the definition of IBS and outlines the range of symptoms that can occur as part of this condition. It covers some of the other gut and brain conditions that often co-occur with IBS, as well as the various ways IBS can affect your quality of life.

Defining IBS

REMEMBER

IBS is a condition defined by digestive symptoms that result from disordered gut-brain interaction. The core symptoms of IBS (occurring in the absence of other conditions that could cause the symptoms) are as follows:

>> **Abdominal pain** that's related to bowel movements

>> **Abnormal bowel movements**, either more or less often than normal (with normal ranging from three times per day to three times per week) or with a different appearance than normal (either loose and watery or hard and lumpy)

Bloating (a feeling of fullness) or *distension* (visible expansion of your belly) often accompanies the pain and abnormal bowel movements of IBS. Doctors use a classification system developed by an organization called the Rome Foundation as the criteria for diagnosing IBS (see the sidebar "Looking to Rome for answers"). The diagnosis is made by confirming the presence of the telltale symptoms while also ruling out other conditions that may cause similar symptoms. (Turn to Chapter 5 for more on getting a diagnosis.)

A key feature of IBS is the absence of physical damage to the digestive tract — so the digestive organs of someone with IBS may look identical to those of someone without IBS. For this reason, IBS was long known as a *functional* disorder, which means it arises from a change in how a body system works (functions) rather than from a physical cause that can be directly measured. Today, functional gastrointestinal (GI) disorders are more accurately called *disorders of gut-brain interaction* (DGBIs; see "Shifting from functional disorders to disorders of gut-brain interaction," later in this chapter, for more on this change).

Over many decades, researchers have tried to find some biological measure that reliably distinguishes people with IBS from those without the condition. No single parameter has so far been shown to reliably identify IBS. See Chapter 3 for biological changes that are seen in some groups of people with IBS.

As researchers studying IBS over the years have learned, despite common symptoms showing up on the surface, people with IBS have very different and complex factors contributing to those symptoms. (You can read more about these factors in Chapters 3 and 4.)

For now, IBS is a catchall category for the main symptoms of abdominal pain and altered bowel movements, and may or may not include bloating, distension, and other symptoms. The section "Understanding IBS Symptoms," later in this chapter, explains the range of digestive symptoms that people with IBS typically experience.

LOOKING TO ROME FOR ANSWERS

For gastroenterologists, the Rome Foundation is not unlike Rome to Catholics: the seat of ultimate wisdom and guidance. The Rome Foundation is a nonprofit scientific organization that drives forward the scientific and clinical understanding of all DGBIs, including IBS. The organization's roots extend back to 1984, when a packed-out international symposium on IBS prompted a group of gastroenterologists to establish working teams to answer some of the questions about IBS and other DGBIs that weren't currently addressed in the scientific literature. In 1988, some of the involved experts formed a committee to establish diagnostic criteria for IBS, which they published shortly thereafter. Through the 1990s and early 2000s, the expert teams reviewed and revised these "gold standard" criteria for diagnosing IBS through a series of publications known as Rome I, Rome II, and Rome III. They officially established the Rome Foundation in 1996, around the time of publication of Rome II. The diagnostic criteria called Rome IV were published in 2016, with Rome V set for 2026. The organization is active today and has been the leading force in moving the research forward and legitimizing IBS throughout the world.

Shifting from functional disorders to disorders of gut-brain interaction

The workings of the digestive tract (see Chapter 4) are so complex and mysterious that they often go awry without any measurable physical cause. Such conditions have long been known in the medical community as functional GI disorders. IBS may be the most famous of these disorders, but the overall category of functional GI disorders is broad and includes functional abdominal pain, functional dyspepsia (indigestion), functional heartburn, and more.

Language tends to shape how people react to a disorder. The problem with calling all of these disorders "functional" was that it put them in contrast with disorders that can be directly tied to a clear physical or chemical problem in the body, with the latter seeming more tangible. The false dichotomy between physical and functional disorders implied that functional disorders were somehow less legitimate. Even though functional disorders are very real to the affected people and to the doctors who hear about certain patterns of symptoms over and over, some people were tempted to conclude that IBS arose from distress or nervousness — or even believed, regrettably, that the affected person was making it all up (see the sidebar "Nothing to see here").

Realizing that the functional moniker was standing in the way of progress, a group of experts proposed that functional disorders be renamed *disorders of gut-brain interaction* (DGBIs). The shift was initiated in 2016 with the publication of new criteria (called Rome IV) for diagnosing IBS and related disorders. This term is currently considered the proper category for IBS and other GI disorders without a physical cause, better reflecting the current scientific knowledge and helping reduce the stigma of IBS around the world.

REMEMBER

Although you may still hear healthcare professionals refer to IBS as a functional disorder, the category of DGBIs is gaining acceptance and is more consistent with researchers' evolving understanding of the multiple processes that work together to determine the symptoms that show up with these GI disorders.

NOTHING TO SEE HERE

In the novel *Dracula* by Bram Stoker, Professor Van Helsing says, "It is the fault of our science that it wants to explain all, and if it explain not, then it says there is nothing to explain." This description has (unfortunately) been true of the study of IBS in previous decades. The lack of an observable structural problem in the digestive tract led some doctors over the years to deny that people with IBS had a legitimate disorder.

In 1892, around the time when the story of *Dracula* is set, a Canadian doctor named William Osler described IBS-like symptoms occurring without damage to the gut wall, and called the affected patients "hysterical, hypochondriac, or depressed." Along these lines, many of the medical writings about IBS-like symptoms before the 1970s were remarkably dismissive and stigmatizing, reflecting a false assumption that body disorders and brain disorders were strictly separate, and further, that brain-related disorders were less defined and somehow less worthy of medical attention. This attitude undoubtedly caused extra pain and suffering for patients of past decades who were dismissed as insane or self-centered. Luckily for individuals with IBS today, the medical community is well aware that IBS is a recognized condition that should be diagnosed and treated appropriately.

Identifying the criteria for diagnosing IBS

To confirm you have IBS, you need a diagnosis from a medical professional — usually a primary-care (family) physician. No single test exists to confirm whether you have IBS. Instead, the doctor makes the diagnosis after gathering a variety of information and assessing whether you meet the current diagnostic criteria for IBS.

REMEMBER

Abdominal pain and changes in the appearance or frequency of bowel movements are the minimum criteria that must be met for IBS. The diagnostic criteria also specify time frames for the symptoms:

>> Abdominal pain must be present at least one day per week over the past three months, coinciding with altered bowel movements.

>> The symptoms must occur for at least six months before they're deemed *chronic* (long-term) and therefore qualify for an IBS diagnosis.

This pattern of symptoms seems to classify people into a distinct group. Symptoms that occur a little less frequently than specified don't qualify you for the IBS diagnosis, so in that case you may be said to have "IBS-like symptoms."

Importantly, any other conditions that could cause the symptoms must be ruled out before you definitively receive an IBS diagnosis. (See Chapter 5 for more details on the process of receiving a diagnosis.)

When IBS is diagnosed, the doctor may specify an IBS subcategory based on whether the GI symptoms are predominantly diarrhea, constipation, or a mix of both (see the next section).

Discovering IBS subtypes

REMEMBER

Distinct subtypes of IBS are based on the pattern of bowel movements: constipation (C), diarrhea (D), or mixed constipation and diarrhea (M). The IBS subtypes are as follows:

>> **IBS-C (constipation):** In this type of IBS, which is the most common, bowel movements may be less frequent, and often take the form of hard, lumpy stools.

>> **IBS-D (diarrhea):** This type of IBS is characterized by frequent bowel movements that usually produce loose, liquid stools.

>> **IBS-M (mixed):** This type of IBS shows up as alternating constipation and diarrhea of which more than a quarter of bowel movements are classified as diarrhea, and more than a quarter are constipation.

Sometimes the different subtypes have different treatments, but other times they can be treated with common strategies. You can learn all about IBS treatment in Part 3 of this book.

Seeing how IBS changes over time

IBS is a *chronic relapsing-remitting* condition, so by definition, the symptoms of IBS may disappear for a short time but return again and again despite your best attempts to ward them off. But can you expect your IBS to stay exactly the same over time, or to change in some ways?

REMEMBER

Some people with IBS experience periods of time without any symptoms. These periods of remission can last for weeks, months, or even years. But for the most part, people with IBS have to accept the fact that their bowel movements may be normal and they may be free of pain for a brief glorious time, although never for an extended period of time.

Even when IBS symptoms are present continually without remission, the way they show up may change over time. Here are some of the ways the symptoms may shift:

>> Symptoms may be more severe sometimes and milder at other times.

>> Symptoms may be very frequent sometimes and occasional at other times.

>> Different symptoms may be added to the mix.

A sudden increase in symptoms for a period of time may be called a *flare* or *flare-up*. Changes between one IBS subtype and another have sometimes been documented in scientific studies. Around one-third of people with IBS may change their subtype, with IBS-M often becoming a different subtype. A shift from IBS-D to IBS-C may occur, but rarely the other way around. New symptoms may occur at times, but if you have existing IBS and you experience new symptoms past age 40, talk with a healthcare professional in case further investigation is required.

In very rare cases — perhaps in 2 percent of people with confirmed IBS — the condition goes away permanently. But complete disappearance of IBS is extremely uncommon. If you have IBS, you should expect to live with it the rest of your life, even if you're lucky enough to experience periods of time where the symptoms taper off or aren't as severe as usual.

Understanding IBS Symptoms

This section lists the range of symptoms that may be part of your IBS experience and flags the less typical symptoms that may be a sign of some other disorder. When IBS occurs with another disorder, sorting out which symptoms are directly a result of the IBS can be a challenging puzzle for you and your doctor to solve. (Turn to Chapter 5 for information on how to differentiate between IBS and other conditions.)

Unsurprisingly, the core symptoms that occur with IBS — abdominal pain, abnormal bowel movements, and sometimes bloating or distension — happen in the GI tract. But in addition to these symptoms that bond together everyone with IBS, other GI symptoms can occur. This section lists the most common symptoms seen in people with IBS.

Abdominal pain

Abdominal pain or discomfort is an unwanted sensation that you feel anywhere in your belly region (between your ribs and your pelvis). It's really this pain that clinches the IBS diagnosis.

The pain can show up in different ways at different times. For example, it may be:

>> Sharp or dull/crampy

>> Located in one place or felt all over your abdominal region (perhaps even extending to your back or chest)

>> Severe (preventing you from doing your normal activities) or mild

Often the pain comes and goes, coinciding with changes in your bowel movements. It may be relieved for a short or long period of time after you have a bowel movement or pass gas. Many people with IBS report that the pain increases after eating, but it may also increase when they haven't eaten for a long time. On the extreme end of the pain scale, some people with IBS who have given birth say their IBS pain is worse than labor pain.

WARNING

The following types of pain are *not* typical in IBS and should prompt a visit to a healthcare professional:

>> Abdominal pain that wakes you up at night

>> Continuous pain with no breaks, even after a bowel movement

>> Pain associated with rectal bleeding, vomiting, or weight loss

>> Pain so severe you have difficulty moving, eating, or drinking

Bloating and distension

The next time your belly looks and feels balloon-like, just search the hashtag #bloated on social media. You'll know with certainty you're not alone when you scroll through the dozens and dozens of photographs showing off side views of distended bellies.

Bloating and distension are besties, usually found together. But there's a difference between them: *Bloating* is a feeling of your belly being full and tight, and *distension* is the visible expansion of your abdominal region. Even though people tend to use *bloating* as the catchall term, bloating is really something you *feel* and distension is something you *see*.

Bloating and/or distension are experienced by 80 percent to 90 percent of people with IBS from time to time. People with the IBS-C subtype may be more certain to experience it than people with IBS-D. Bloating and distension may get worse after eating, and they may make you constantly feel like you need to pass gas. If you do pass gas or have a bowel movement, your bloating and distension may be relieved temporarily.

WARNING

Here's what's *not* so typical for IBS and should get you to visit a healthcare professional:

>> Recurrent bloating and distension that don't seem tied to your eating pattern in any way

>> Bloating and distension accompanied by severe abdominal pain, fever, or vomiting, and without a bowel movement or passage of gas

Borborygmi

Borborygmi are rumbling or gurgling noises that originate in the digestive tract from the movement of food, fluid, or gases. Although these noises are not considered a core symptom of IBS, and they frequently occur in completely healthy people, they can often cause embarrassment and, thus, interfere with quality of life.

Constipation

Constipation happens when you have infrequent or effortful bowel movements, with the stools tending to be hard and lumpy. The medical definition of *constipation* includes various symptoms:

>> Straining or taking a long time to pass stools

>> Hard stools

>> Infrequent bowel movements (less than every three days)

>> A continual feeling of incomplete emptying of the bowels

WARNING

Individuals with IBS-C or IBS-M may experience these symptoms regularly. However, if these symptoms of constipation come on suddenly and don't go away, see a healthcare professional.

Diarrhea

Diarrhea is identified by the following symptoms:

>> More frequent bowel movements (perhaps more than three times per day, or just more frequently than normal for you)

>> Loose or liquid stools

>> A sense of urgency when you have a bowel movement

For a bowel movement to be classified as diarrhea, you must have either liquid stools or an increased frequency of bowel movements.

TECHNICAL STUFF

Technically, the classification of diarrhea is based on the volume of stool passed — more than 7 ounces (200 grams) per day — but most doctors will be happy to take your word for it and won't demand quantifiable proof of your daily stool volume.

Diarrhea is very common in people with IBS, and it may occur soon after eating.

WARNING

It's common for people with IBS-D to feel a sense of urgency, as if they may have an accident, and occasionally they may lose control. If you experience *incontinence* (loss of control of your bowels) more than in rare circumstances, make sure to talk with a healthcare professional about it. Other symptoms that signal something other than IBS are:

>> Persistent diarrhea with no breaks

>> Diarrhea that wakes you up at night

>> Blood in the stool

>> Diarrhea that occurs when fasting

>> Diarrhea that lasts for several days and is accompanied by fever or vomiting

WARNING

With frequent or severe diarrhea, you run the risk of becoming dehydrated. If you have signs of dehydration, such as infrequent urination, a dry mouth, or a feeling of lightheadedness, sip water or use a rehydration solution right away.

Intestinal gas and burping

Digestion is gassy work. The microorganisms living in your digestive tract are mostly responsible for the amount and type of gases produced in response to the foods you eat. These gases (hydrogen, carbon dioxide, sulfur, and sometimes methane) need to go somewhere, so after a portion is absorbed into the lining of the colon, the rest is expelled (an occurrence called *flatulence*).

At the other end, *burping* or *belching* (technically known as *eructation*) is typically caused by swallowing excess air that needs to be released. Carbonated drinks are one obvious culprit. But without realizing it, you may swallow more air when you eat or drink quickly, chew gum, suck on a candy, smoke or vape, or talk while you're eating. Other things that can cause burping include stomach inflammation or infection, and bacterial overgrowth in the upper GI tract.

People with IBS often experience increased gas and sometimes burping. Passage of gas is often associated with temporary relief of abdominal pain.

WARNING

See a healthcare professional if:

>> You suddenly experience much more gas or burping than normal even though you haven't changed your diet.

>> You experience excessive burping or gas along with vomiting.

Other gastrointestinal symptoms

Other GI symptoms can occur as part of the IBS spectrum. Another common symptom is *nausea*, an uneasy feeling that you may vomit, which you may feel in your stomach or the back of your throat. Vomiting may or may not actually occur.

WARNING

Other symptoms are *not* typical for IBS, and are alarm symptoms that should prompt you to contact a healthcare professional to investigate urgently:

>> Blood in your stools

>> Black, tarry stools

>> Unexplained, rapid weight loss

>> Fever with GI symptoms

>> Recurrent vomiting

>> Difficulty swallowing food

Exploring Common Conditions That Tend to Occur with IBS

Even though IBS is a distinct condition that can exist on its own, researchers have found that people with IBS have a higher chance of being diagnosed with some other conditions. The typically co-occurring conditions can originate in the gut, in the brain, or elsewhere. Some of these conditions may interact with IBS, making the symptoms better or worse over time.

These conditions commonly pair with IBS, although they can appear separately, too. Some of them share the same predisposing factors or underlying mechanisms as IBS. A carefully considered diagnosis is an important first step to determine whether you have something going on in addition to IBS. Details on the process of diagnosis are covered in Chapter 5.

Gut conditions that may co-occur with IBS

REMEMBER

IBS is a condition defined by gut symptoms, but that doesn't mean every gut symptom you have is attributable to IBS. Knowing whether you have other conditions besides IBS is important because it may shape the treatment approach you take. Here are some other gut-related conditions that can crop up alongside IBS.

Food reactions

An adverse food reaction involves unwanted symptoms that are consistent and predictable after eating a certain type of food.

Food reactions fall into two general categories, depending on whether the immune system is involved:

>> A **food allergy** is a type of reaction that triggers an immune response that causes inflammation and damage to body tissues. The most typical kind of allergy, such as a peanut allergy, occurs when a food triggers production of *antibodies* (proteins that fight substances the body deems harmful), causing the release of proinflammatory chemicals that cause symptoms such as itching, swelling, and sometimes difficulty breathing — meaning that the reaction can be life-threatening. This type of allergy is rare in adults (but more common in children), and it's unlikely to be the cause of food-related symptoms in adults with IBS.

>> A **food intolerance** or **food sensitivity** is discomfort caused by difficulty digesting a particular food. For example, if your body doesn't produce enough of the enzyme necessary to digest lactose (a sugar found in dairy products), you experience symptoms when you consume lactose and you're considered lactose intolerant. These food reactions are not triggered by the immune system and are not life-threatening.

Diagnosing these conditions typically involves a thorough medical history, experimenting with diet, and, in some cases, specialized testing. Food reactions can be difficult to pinpoint without systematically eliminating certain foods. However, extreme elimination diets can cause further health problems, including nutritional deficiencies, so the ideal situation is to explore food reactions under the supervision of a registered dietitian. Find further details in Chapter 7.

Histamine intolerance

Histamine is a type of chemical that is naturally produced by your body and is also present in some foods. Histamine intolerance happens when the body can't break down histamine fast enough, causing it to build up and cause symptoms. A wide range of symptoms can occur as a result: bloating, gas, diarrhea, or constipation, as well as symptoms outside the digestive system, such as nasal congestion, shortness of breath, and sneezing. It may also cause skin symptoms such as itching, redness, hives, and swelling. The symptoms can closely mimic an allergy but do not involve the immune system.

Histamine is naturally found in various foods, such as seafood, avocados, nuts, milk, legumes, and certain fruits such as bananas. It's also released by bacteria (such as lactobacilli) during the process of fermentation so high amounts of histamines tend to be present in fermented foods and beverages such as aged cheese, chocolate, kimchi, and kombucha.

Diagnosing histamine intolerance can be difficult because the symptoms overlap with other conditions, and no specific tests can confirm it. A dietitian can help you explore whether you may have a histamine intolerance. A low-histamine diet may help treat histamine intolerance, and can be tried for a two-week period under the guidance of a dietitian knowledgeable in this area. If your symptoms persist after trying a low-histamine diet, medical therapies may be warranted.

Small intestinal bacterial overgrowth

A sparse community of microorganisms normally lives in your small intestine (in contrast with the more complex community in your large intestine), performing essential digestive functions (see Chapter 4). Small intestinal bacterial overgrowth (SIBO, pronounced see-bo) is a disruption in both the number and type of small intestinal microorganisms — so too many microbes of the wrong type proliferate in the upper digestive tract, causing abdominal pain, diarrhea, bloating and distension, along with other symptoms that can look very much like IBS.

In the medical community, some debate exists over whether SIBO should be considered one of the underlying causes of IBS or a separate condition. For the purposes of this book, we consider SIBO a condition that is identified on its own, separately from IBS. SIBO may be identified using a noninvasive breath test, but the test is rarely used now in clinical practice. Instead, if SIBO is suspected, the doctor may recommend antibiotic treatment and then assess how you respond. Some studies have found that treating SIBO seems to correlate with the improvement of IBS symptoms in general.

Brain conditions that co-occur with IBS

Several brain-related conditions tend to occur with IBS. Studies estimate that more than half of people with IBS have an accompanying psychological condition such as anxiety or depression. Because of the disordered gut-brain communication in IBS, affected individuals are three times more likely to have anxiety or depression than people in the general population.

Anxiety or depression (or both) that occur with IBS have a particularly important impact on quality of life, sometimes interfering with the ability to work and carry out daily activities. In addition, people who have anxiety or depression tend to have more severe IBS symptoms due to the vicious cycle of gut-brain disruption (see Chapter 4). When people with an IBS diagnosis are followed over time, researchers often find that anxiety, depression, or both often emerge at some point.

Anxiety

Clinical anxiety disorders, characterized by persistent or uncontrollable feelings of worry that may interfere with daily life, are known to co-occur with several GI disorders, including IBS. Estimates of anxiety among people with IBS are difficult to obtain because many people experience anxiety-like symptoms without seeking a formal diagnosis. However, various studies estimate between 16 percent and 38 percent of people with IBS also have anxiety.

If you think you may have anxiety, it's best to seek the opinion of a healthcare professional so the condition can be diagnosed and treated appropriately, avoiding further exacerbation of IBS symptoms.

Depression

Major depressive disorder is a mood disorder in which people experience chronic feelings of sadness and a loss of interest in the activities of daily life. Depression often co-occurs with GI symptoms, with constipation frequently accompanying it. According to scientific studies, around 30 percent of people with IBS also have depression — but many cases of depression also go undiagnosed.

When you have IBS, a proper diagnosis of depression is key, enabling you to discuss various treatment options and maintain a handle on both the gut and the brain symptoms.

Migraines

Migraine is a type of headache characterized by bouts of throbbing and pulsating pain on one side of the head, which last anywhere from a few hours to three days. The pain is caused by the activation of nerve fibers in the central nervous system. It may start gradually and build in intensity.

Individuals with IBS appear more likely to have migraines than the general population. Migraines occur more often in women and in people who have both IBS and anxiety.

Other brain-related conditions

Several other brain-related conditions seem to have a higher-than-average chance of existing in people diagnosed with IBS. These conditions include:

>> Post-traumatic stress disorder

>> Sleep impairments

>> Parkinson's disease (which involves gut symptoms that arise because of different factors from the ones in IBS)

So far, scientists have not confirmed that IBS is part of what causes these conditions. Research is ongoing to discover whether common biological mechanisms exist for IBS and other brain-related disorders.

Other conditions that co-occur with IBS

Several other conditions that are not based in the gut or the brain tend to co-occur with IBS. The two main conditions are chronic fatigue syndrome and fibromyalgia.

Chronic fatigue syndrome

Chronic fatigue syndrome (CFS), also known as *myalgic encephalomyelitis* (ME), causes severe fatigue that worsens with exercise and doesn't fully improve with rest. This extreme tiredness is often accompanied by cognitive dysfunction, debilitating pain, and lack of proper sleep.

Individuals with IBS have a greater chance of experiencing CFS than the general population. Finding a diagnosis of CFS can require persistence, so you may need to advocate for yourself in a calm and kind manner. Fortunately, awareness and knowledge about this condition is increasing within the medical community.

Fibromyalgia

Fibromyalgia is a chronic pain disorder that involves widespread body pains as well as muscle and joint stiffness, insomnia, fatigue, mood problems, headaches, difficulty concentrating, and GI symptoms.

The occurrence of fibromyalgia is significantly higher in people with IBS compared to the general population. The two conditions share symptoms and are frequently co-diagnosed. Very commonly, people diagnosed with IBS and fibromyalgia together experience mood or psychological symptoms as well.

Being Aware of How IBS Affects Your Quality of Life

When you have IBS, caring for your grumpy gut can take up a lot of your time and energy. You may devote extra time to strategizing about how to avoid provoking symptoms, which takes your mind off the things you'd rather be thinking about. Your symptoms may stand in the way of going where you want to go and doing what you want to do. Studies show that IBS is associated with both *absenteeism* (regular absence from work or school) and *presenteeism* (lower productivity when you're present there).

Quality of life (QoL) is a measure of well-being that takes into consideration both positive and negative factors about your life at a specific point in time. Your QoL is your subjective feeling about your overall enjoyment and comfort given the people and environment around you. Many factors contribute to this perception, including both facts about your life (such as your income) and personal factors (such as your personality and how you think people react to you). Researchers have surveys for measuring a person's health-related QoL and overall QoL.

Studies show that IBS can have disproportionate effects on QoL. In fact, people with IBS often rate their QoL as lower than people with more serious diseases such as heart failure, diabetes, or end-stage kidney disease.

Several main aspects of living with IBS may threaten to take away from your QoL: how you limit your daily activities, your experiences of pain, and feeling held back in your life and career.

HOW STIGMA AFFECTS QUALITY OF LIFE

Almost all people with IBS have likely seen evidence of *stigma*, or other peoples' negative perceptions, at some point in time. It could be a boss frustrated by your need to manage your symptoms, a friend who makes a hurtful comment when you have to cancel a plan, or a family member who loudly opines on what they think really ails you. Stigma is hard to avoid because, although you can control your own reaction to your IBS, you can't control other people's reactions. Studies show that when you experience stigma related to your IBS, you tend to rate your quality of life as being lower. Fortunately, at this point in history, IBS stigma (while still present) seems to be at an all-time low. IBS awareness days prompt people to wear periwinkle ribbons and illuminate stadiums with purple lights, and celebrities and social media influencers are loud and proud about their IBS. With any luck, experiences of stigma will decrease in frequency over the coming years. In the meantime, see Chapter 13 for some tips on minimizing the effects of stigma and maximizing how you thrive with IBS.

Restricting your activities

When you decide not to do something because of how you anticipate your IBS will affect that activity, your QoL may be affected in a negative way. This activity restriction can happen on a daily scale, such as declining to visit someone's house for book club, or on a longer time scale, as in the case of Allison missing out on a yearly girls' weekend that would've helped her create great memories with her friends. Changing your activities allows you to implement better self-care, but the trade-off is that you may miss out on happy moments and things you enjoy.

Getting a handle on your symptoms through appropriate treatment may help you increase your QoL by allowing you to go ahead with activities and not be held back by your symptoms. Part 3 of this book discusses a variety of treatment options.

Experiencing pain

One of the key symptoms of IBS, abdominal pain, can interfere with your everyday activities by making you lose concentration or making movements uncomfortable.

Even if you're not held back from doing what you want, pain can get in the way of feeling light and energetic. And when you're constantly dealing with pain, it's bound to put a damper on your mood.

Management of pain in IBS is a key focus of some treatment strategies. If your pain is the predominant symptom getting in the way of your wellness, talk to a healthcare professional about how to address that aspect of your IBS.

Meeting goals in your life and career

People with IBS sometimes report that their QoL is affected by what's happening in the bigger picture of their life — where they're going overall in their life and career. They may feel that the practicalities of IBS are holding them back from reaching their goals. Even when day-to-day life is relatively comfortable and manageable, some people wish they could push themselves to do more.

REMEMBER

The good news is that you can be empowered through some of the strategies in this book to manage the daily symptoms of IBS in a way that will enable you, over time, to get closer to where you want to go. See Part 3 of this book for effective IBS management options, and Chapter 13 for a wealth of information on maintaining your QoL with IBS.

Chapter **3**

Discovering Who Gets IBS and Why

Think about all the people you may see when you're out in public: the person strolling by with a dog on a leash, the cashier at the grocery store, the person operating the crane on a construction site, the group of people sitting and talking at a coffee shop. Chances are, some of these people have irritable bowel syndrome (IBS). But we can almost guarantee none of them has a badge on their lapel announcing "I have IBS."

Even among the circle of people you know pretty well, you may not be able to tell which of them are living with IBS. Some people just aren't inclined to talk about their gut symptoms, or they may have had negative experiences when disclosing their gut problems in the past. You may not ever know that digestive troubles are the reason they need to decline an invitation or cancel plans.

So, you may not have a true sense of how many people in the world actually have IBS. The condition is surprisingly common, and chances are, a good number of the people you come into contact with every day are living with it.

This chapter walks you through the range of people who can get IBS and the risk factors that make an IBS diagnosis more likely. We fill you in on what doctors and researchers know about the underlying causes of the condition, including the possible role of the gut microbes that live in your digestive tract. We also outline some actions people who don't already have the condition can take to help prevent it.

Identifying Who's Affected by IBS

Before the 1980s, stereotypes of the typical IBS patient abounded in the medical community.

REMEMBER

Today doctors know that no restriction exists on the type of person who can experience IBS. The condition can affect a wide variety of people from all walks of life, and it can first emerge at different times in their lives.

Nevertheless, some groups of people or people with certain habits and exposures are more likely to get IBS. This section covers the statistics on how common IBS is and the factors about a person and their experiences that make an IBS diagnosis more likely.

How common IBS is

Every day, people are diagnosed with IBS in doctors' offices all over the world. But figuring out how many people have IBS overall is surprisingly difficult for researchers. The investigations that have tried to discover the *prevalence* of IBS (or how widespread it is) in the general population have come up with varying results.

TECHNICAL STUFF

Here are some of the reasons that estimating the prevalence of IBS is difficult:

>> Not everyone wants to share information about their digestive health with researchers or clinicians because of stigma or other personal factors.

>> Some people have symptoms that meet the criteria for IBS but don't have an official diagnosis.

>> Some people may not seek the help of medical professionals at all — they feel they can manage the symptoms on their own.

>> Researchers sometimes have difficulty accessing the health information that would allow them to determine if someone has IBS or IBS-like symptoms.

Here's what we know: Conditions that are part of the overarching category for IBS — *disorders of gut-brain interaction* (DGBIs) — are very common overall. A study of more than 70,000 people across 24 countries found that approximately 40 percent of people met the criteria for at least one DGBI.

IBS is the most common type of DGBI. The global estimate of how many people have IBS is around 11 percent. However, most cases of IBS remain undiagnosed at any point in time, so the true prevalence may be higher. In the United States, researchers have determined that around 6 percent of people have an official IBS diagnosis and about 15 percent have symptoms that could qualify as IBS.

The prevalence of IBS varies in different countries. One global analysis from 2012 reported varying rates of people that met the criteria for IBS, from a low of around 3 percent in France to higher rates of 17 percent in Brazil, 18 percent in Canada, 28 percent in Pakistan, and 32 percent in Nigeria.

These numbers may not be static over time, however. For example, a 2024 news article in the United Kingdom (UK) reported on healthcare data showing that new IBS diagnoses had reached a ten-year high. Diagnoses of IBS had dipped briefly for both men and women in 2020, coinciding with the COVID-19 pandemic (likely due to fewer people accessing medical services), before starting to climb to new highs. This increase in diagnoses is expected to result in a higher overall prevalence in the UK. Cases of IBS continue to increase in some other countries as well.

Some of the apparent increase in IBS prevalence may be chalked up to better awareness, in part because of greater advocacy from patient organizations, shining a light on IBS and designating awareness weeks or months. In addition, many people hear about IBS on social media and are more willing to seek out advice from a healthcare professional. But beyond this increased engagement around IBS, the condition may be increasing across the population. Researchers haven't yet identified a specific reason for this increase.

Who's at risk for IBS

Researchers are not able to predict exactly who will develop IBS, but over time, they've identified some risk factors that make a diagnosis more likely.

Here is the list of factors that appear to give someone a higher chance of developing IBS:

>> **Sex:** People assigned female at birth have a much higher risk of IBS, with the condition being twice or even three times as common in females as it is in males.

>> **Age:** Unlike the majority of chronic diseases, which are more likely to develop with age, younger people have a higher risk of developing IBS. The most common age for IBS to emerge is in early adulthood, and it rarely emerges for the first time in people over the age of 50.

>> **Existing depression or anxiety:** If you have a diagnosis of depression or anxiety without gut symptoms, you're more likely to develop IBS over time.

>> **Adverse childhood events:** Traumatic events that happen in childhood — such as abuse, mental illness, or domestic violence — are connected with developing several health problems later in life. Studies have found that these adverse events at a young age give you a higher chance of developing IBS.

>> **Occurrence of a gut infection:** A typical case of a sudden gastrointestinal infection caused by harmful microorganisms (for example, food poisoning) involves vomiting and gut symptoms such as diarrhea. Experiencing this kind of infection for a few days greatly increases your risk for developing IBS. According to some estimates, a whopping 10 percent to 30 percent of people who experience a sudden-onset gut infection develop IBS-like symptoms (abdominal pain with diarrhea, constipation, and/or bloating) that persist for months or years, or that never go away.

>> **Taking antibiotics:** Large population studies have shown that people who took one or more courses of antibiotics in previous years tended to have a greater chance of developing IBS.

>> **Stress:** IBS is more likely to occur if you experience a sudden increase in your perceived stress levels or a major new source of stress in your life. The stress you feel can be for many different reasons: physical difficulties, financial pressures, tough social and emotional situations, or other factors.

>> **Smoking:** If you're currently a smoker, or if you used to be a smoker, you have an increased chance of developing IBS.

>> **Pesticide exposure:** Emerging evidence points to the idea that people who live in areas with heavy pesticide exposure are more likely to develop IBS.

>> **What you eat and drink:** No specific food causes IBS, but you have an increased risk if your diet fits a Western diet pattern, consisting of a high intake of sugar, processed foods, and saturated fats, with a lack of fiber. High alcohol intake is also associated with a greater chance of having IBS.

>> **How much sleep you get:** Researchers have determined that people who fail to get seven or more hours of quality sleep per night have a higher risk of IBS.

>> **Physical activity:** If you don't get vigorous exercise regularly, you're increasing your risk of developing IBS.

>> **Family history of IBS:** If you have a first-degree relative with IBS, you're more likely to develop the condition yourself. But interestingly, researchers have not found specific genes linked to IBS, so it's not considered a genetic condition. One genetic study of more than 250,000 people with IBS found that certain genes may predispose people to both IBS and anxiety/mood disorders simultaneously. This finding underscores the common underlying origins of both gut-related and brain-related problems linked to IBS.

Some of these risk factors you can't do anything about, but others you can — emphasizing the power of lifestyle to control your risk for IBS.

REMEMBER

Risk factors are not the same as the underlying causes of IBS, and they don't determine with 100 percent certainty whether you'll get IBS. Plenty of people check multiple boxes on the list of risk factors and still don't develop IBS. Think of risk factors as being somehow directly or indirectly linked to the root causes of IBS (in a manner that's not yet understood) — so they may decrease your chances of developing IBS if you modify them.

IBS AFTER INFECTION

A sudden gut infection, such as food poisoning or infectious diarrhea, is not the most pleasant experience. As if the intense vomiting and diarrhea weren't bad enough, a little-known side effect of gut infections is the possibility of developing lasting IBS-like symptoms or full-blown IBS after the infection goes away, a condition called *post-infectious IBS*.

In 1945, when World War II was over, doctors documented persistent gastrointestinal symptoms in some of the soldiers and sailors who had previously contracted dysentery while on duty, even though the pathogenic microbes had long been cleared from their guts. The Scottish doctor G.T. Stewart wrote in the *British Medical Journal* that the observed lingering diarrhea may have been due to long-term changes in the intestinal microorganisms — a theory that is today backed by increasing evidence.

Post-infectious IBS has been increasingly documented since the 1940s. In one high-profile incident known as the Walkerton water tragedy, contamination of the drinking water supply in Walkerton, Canada, in 2000 led to nearly half of the town's residents being infected with pathogenic *E. coli* and experiencing bloody diarrhea, vomiting, cramps, and fever. Around 2,300 people became ill, and at least 7 people died. After the terrible crisis, researchers kept tabs on people in the town. After two to three years, around 28 percent of the participants who had gotten ill from the drinking water met the criteria for IBS. After eight years, this number was reduced to 15 percent. Finally, eight years after the infection, the risk factors for IBS in the town mirrored the risk factors for IBS in general: being a woman, being young, and having existing anxiety or depression. In addition, IBS had tended to persist longer in those who had fever or significant weight loss during the initial infection.

CHALLENGING IBS STEREOTYPES: THE "HOT GIRLS HAVE IBS" BILLBOARDS

If you were driving down a highway in Los Angeles, California, sometime in October 2021, you may have done a double take when you saw a bold pink billboard with yellow stars, featuring the bold phrase "Hot Girls Have IBS." The billboard was part of an ad campaign for BelliWelli, a company selling IBS-friendly cookies — and it clearly tapped into the important concept that IBS may affect the people you least expect, and it may be hidden behind a person's put-together external image. The ad campaign immediately went viral. People took pictures of the billboard and posted them on social media, disclosing their own gut issues. Posts about the billboards generated millions of views and a nearly endless feed of comments. BelliWelli's sales shot up — but more important, the campaign helped disrupt stereotypes and empowered the image-conscious crowd to talk about their gut problems with less shame.

Recognizing What Causes IBS

Many people who currently have IBS weren't born with it. But somewhere along the line, it seems, their body flipped a switch and started to manifest recurring digestive symptoms. How this switch gets flipped is a question that scientists don't quite have the answer to, but as with many chronic conditions, the processes leading to IBS probably start a long time before you meet the criteria for diagnosis. In this section, we describe the emerging clues as to the causes of IBS.

Overall, the current research paints a picture of IBS as a mismatch between your outer environment and your inner environment. Whereas your outer environment encompasses everything outside your body (such as your geographical location, your home, and the people you interact with), your inner environment includes all the biological processes that help keep your body working normally. Think about how a panda bear has different biology from a polar bear. They aren't expected to thrive equally well in an arctic ecosystem. Similarly, you can think about IBS as your outer environment being out of sync with what your gut-brain biology is equipped to handle. Put simply, both external and internal factors contribute to the emergence of IBS.

Gaining insights into how IBS arises

IBS is a cluster of outward symptoms that has a variety of root causes. On a biological level, IBS is complex, with no single cause being identified by the world's best researchers and doctors. However, emerging observations are starting to show some of the biological changes that are triggered in subgroups of people with IBS:

>> **Disrupted gut-brain interactions:** The normal two-way channels of gut-brain communication (see Chapter 4) are nerve stimulation, the immune system, and chemical messengers. These modes of communication may be faulty in IBS, causing erratic signals to travel between the gut and the brain, and vice versa. The disrupted signaling may be either top-down (with the brain signaling in ways that affect the gut's pain sensitivity or *motility* [how food and fluids move through the digestive tract]) or bottom-up (with the nerves far away from the brain being oversensitive and activating the brain's pain centers).

>> **Abnormal gastrointestinal motility:** Digestive tract motility tends to be irregular in people with IBS. When motility is too fast or too slow, someone with IBS can experience either diarrhea or constipation, as well as cramping, bloating, or abdominal pain. The underlying cause may be an abnormality in the part of the nervous system that controls the gut's muscle contractions, or a dysfunction in hormone or neuron signaling.

>> **Increased sensitivity to pain in the digestive tract:** Scientists have devised experiments to test how people with IBS experience sensations in their digestive tracts. In one type of experiment, researchers stretch the digestive tract tissues by inserting a balloon into the rectum and filling it with gradually increasing amounts of air. People with IBS feel pain more often and at lower balloon air volumes than people without IBS, which is called *visceral hypersensitivity*. A variety of normal gut sensations cause pain in people with visceral hypersensitivity. Different studies have found that anywhere from 30 percent to 90 percent of people with IBS show this hypersensitivity.

>> **A more permeable gut barrier:** Normally the gut barrier seals off the digestive tract from the rest of the body and has spaces between cells that can open up, like a venetian blind, to let in essential nutrients. Some groups of people with IBS, primarily those with IBS-D (diarrhea), are shown to have an overly permeable gut barrier. This leaky gut barrier is associated with inflammation, as well as more bowel disturbances and abdominal pain.

>> **Dysregulation of the immune system:** Different patterns of immune cell activation are shown to be present in people with IBS, even though the typical markers of colonic and body-wide inflammation may be normal. Research has identified some inflammatory *cytokines* (molecules that send tissue-healing signals from the immune system) that are increased In subgroups of people with IBS. Low-level body-wide inflammation may also be present.

>> **Pelvic floor dysfunction:** When the muscles of the pelvic floor don't work properly, people have difficulty with proper bowel movements, which may

lead to gastrointestinal symptoms. Dysfunctional pelvic floor muscles are common in people with IBS and may or may not lead to the diagnosis of a separate pelvic floor disorder.

>> **Difficulty digesting or absorbing selected carbohydrates:** Some individuals with IBS have altered chemistry in the small intestine that causes them to improperly absorb certain carbohydrates. These carbohydrates reach the colon, where they're broken down by bacteria to produce gases and water, leading to diarrhea and other symptoms. Alternatively, some people lack the *enzymes* (chemicals) to break down specific carbohydrates such as the lactose in milk, causing digestive symptoms.

>> **Changes in the community of gut microbes:** The community of microbes living in your gut (see Chapter 4) carry out important functions needed for you to maintain your health. Numerous studies have found differences in the types and amounts of microorganisms in the digestive tracts of people with IBS compared to healthy people. However, scientists haven't been able to single out a type of microorganism that is always increased or decreased — instead, the changes in the gut ecosystem tend to look slightly different for each person. New research suggests that the gut microbes may be part of IBS susceptibility: Lifestyle factors such as your diet and sleep may shift your community of gut microbes, which in turn contributes to certain biological effects that lead to the development of IBS symptoms. More research in the years ahead will make these connections clearer.

REMEMBER

Each of these biological changes tends to be present in some groups of people with IBS, but not every change is present in every individual. Plus, the nature of the change (for example, the exact way that the gut microbial community is altered) often varies from one person with IBS to the next. And perhaps most important, these changes are also sometimes seen in disorders besides IBS. So, none of them can currently be used to diagnose IBS. Although no factor from this list can explain every case of IBS, over time scientists may discover that combinations of these factors can provide meaningful targets for IBS interventions.

Preventing IBS

If you have IBS, you may look back on the time before you struggled with pain and other gut symptoms and feel a twinge of nostalgia for those more carefree times. Having digestive upset as a constant companion is not for the faint of heart.

For anyone who doesn't have IBS or IBS-like symptoms — perhaps your siblings or children — it's a good idea to take actions to reduce the chance of developing IBS in the future.

REMEMBER

IBS arises from a complex interplay of factors, both internal and external, so ultimately whether someone gets IBS isn't completely under their control. But anyone can be proactive now in their daily life to decrease their chances of getting IBS.

In a large UK study in the journal *Gut*, which included more than 64,000 people, researchers studied five specific habits for preventing IBS: not smoking, getting good-quality sleep, engaging in regular vigorous physical activity, eating a high-quality diet, and moderating alcohol intake. The more of these habits the participants reported, the less likely they were to develop IBS over the 12 years of the study. People who implemented three to five of these behaviors were able to lower their risk of IBS by more than 40 percent!

TIP

Here are the actions you can take now to lower your risk for developing IBS if you don't currently have it:

>> Avoid infections by practicing good hand hygiene and food safety.

>> Be careful about your use of antibiotics — only use them when necessary and recommended by a healthcare professional.

>> Reduce the stress in your life as much as possible, and develop strategies that help you cope with stress.

>> Don't smoke.

>> Adopt a Mediterranean-style, gut-friendly diet with lots of fresh fruits and vegetables and whole grains, as well as fish/seafood.

>> Limit your consumption of red meat, processed foods with many additives, and sugary foods.

>> Moderate your alcohol intake and avoid binge drinking.

>> Get seven or more hours of quality sleep per night.

>> Stay physically active. Aim for 150 minutes per week of moderate or vigorous exercise.

Based on these factors, if you think you may have a higher risk for IBS, make sure you note any changes in bowel habits over time and discuss them with your doctor.

For more details on the actions that can help keep your gut in tip-top shape while avoiding IBS and related gastrointestinal symptoms, check out the book *Gut Health For Dummies*, by Kristina Campbell (John Wiley & Sons). The book provides guidance on how to implement a gut-friendly diet, with high-fiber recipes that nourish both you and your gut microbes.

MICHAEL'S CASE: WAITING ON THE ECONOMY TO CHANGE

Michael, a 42-year-old man, had a demanding Monday-to-Friday job as a financial consultant. He was divorced with two small children (ages 3 and 5), who he cared for on the weekends. During a particularly bad time for the economy, which was stressful for his firm and led to many difficult conversations with clients, he started to experience moderate to severe abdominal pain that lasted for hours at a stretch. The pain got worse after eating, which led him to skip lunch most days at the office. But after eating his evening meal, the pain tended to return, causing Michael to have difficulty falling asleep at bedtime. Michael was also constipated and typically had a bowel movement only twice a week. He believed that when the economy improved, his stress would dissipate and his symptoms would become milder. Yet a year later, when the stock market was showing signs of strength again and his job had become less difficult, his symptoms remained. At this time, Michael saw his family doctor and received a diagnosis of IBS.

Michael's case illustrates how IBS can emerge during a time of particular stress but may not resolve when the source of stress goes away.

Chapter 4

Understanding How the Gut-Brain Axis Works in IBS

At a basic level, your digestive tract (also called your gastrointestinal tract or your gut) is a long tube that extends from your mouth down to your anus. The digestive tract is well known for what it does best: digest and absorb. It does an excellent job of dealing with everything you consume and extracting the energy you need to keep going.

Even though digestion and absorption are the top jobs for your digestive tract, you'd be mistaken to think of this part of your body as a specialist in only these areas. Your digestive tract has another very important task: communicating constantly back and forth with your brain to keep both your brain and your gut functioning smoothly.

Buckle up for some fascinating, nerdy information in this chapter. First, we cover how digestion works — not only how food moves through the digestive tract, but also the lesser-known factors that are critical for normal digestive function. Then we give you the details on how the gut and the brain communicate with each other under normal circumstances. Finally, we explain how gut-brain communication changes in irritable bowel syndrome (IBS) and how the cycle of stress and gastro-intestinal symptoms can be sustained over time.

Clarifying How Your Gut Works

A duck gliding smoothly over the water is a good representation of how your digestive tract works at the best of times: serene on the surface but paddling its feet energetically underneath. In your gut, the everyday work of digesting a meal seems quiet and orderly when everything is functioning well. But under the surface, many complex interactions must occur at the right times and places to keep everything happening smoothly.

The tube of your digestive tract is assisted by some other organs — your liver, pancreas, and gallbladder — which together make up your digestive system as a whole. These accessory organs supply digestive juices needed for certain purposes.

The digestive system works as a unit to accomplish the following:

>> Breaking down substances mechanically (that is, by physically making the parts smaller), as well as chemically and microbially

>> Absorbing nutrients (including water and micronutrients) through your gut barrier so they can reach the rest of your body and travel to where they're needed

>> Transforming one substance into another that's needed in your body (for example, transforming fiber into molecules called short-chain fatty acids, or SCFAs, which supply energy to your gut)

>> Producing essential vitamins and minerals

>> Removing substances you no longer need

>> Repairing and renewing the intestinal tissues so digestion can continue unhindered

>> Regulating the community of gut microorganisms

In addition to these digestive tasks, the other main function that the digestive system must manage is defense: protecting you from microorganisms and toxins that could harm your body. This function is accomplished by your gut immune system. Only by balancing out the two functions of digestion (letting things in) and defense (keeping things out) is your digestive system able to maintain a stable environment.

When a substance enters your digestive tract, it's not in a fully usable form, nor is it fully integrated into your body yet. The digestive tract sequesters everything inside and only lets out specific components after giving them a security check. The gut barrier controls which components of ingested substances end up being allowed into the body and circulated in the blood, and which ones remain inside the digestive tract to be further processed, or shipped down and out. Figure 4-1 shows the basic structure of the gut barrier.

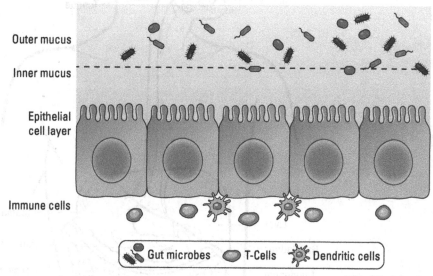

FIGURE 4-1:
The parts of the gut barrier.

This section of the chapter describes the structure of your digestive tract plus the other important but lesser-known systems that are necessary for smooth digestive functioning: the enteric nervous system, gut microorganisms, the immune system, and the enteroendocrine system.

Reviewing the basic structure of your gut

This section takes you on a sightseeing tour of all the major locations in the digestive journey: think "hop-on, hop-off bus tour," but in the digestive tract. Figure 4-2 illustrates the parts of the digestive system.

Oral cavity

The first stop on the digestive tract tour is the *oral cavity,* or mouth. This is where a food or drink first comes into contact with your digestive tract.

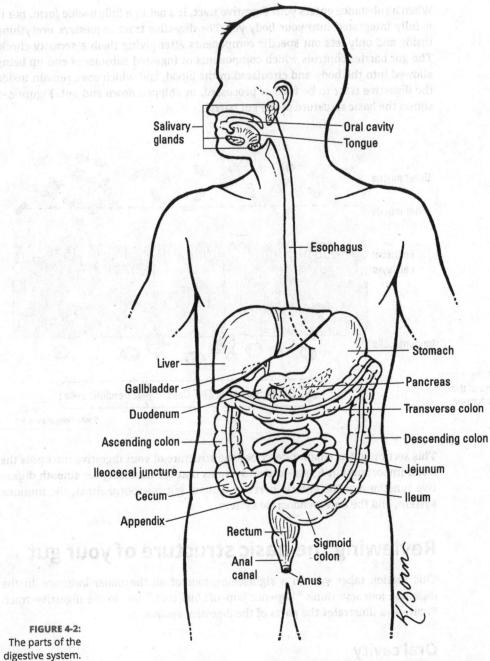

Salivary glands

Oral cavity

Tongue

Esophagus

Stomach

Liver

Pancreas

Gallbladder

Transverse colon

Duodenum

Ascending colon

Descending colon

Ileocecal juncture

Jejunum

Cecum

Ileum

Appendix

Rectum

Sigmoid colon

Anal canal

Anus

K. Born

FIGURE 4-2:
The parts of the
digestive system.

© *John Wiley & Sons, Inc.*

For a larger piece of food, chewing physically breaks it down into smaller pieces. Then saliva, which contains *enzymes* (chemicals that help break things down), mixes with the food and starts the chemical process of digestion: Salivary amylase breaks down starches, and lingual lipase breaks down triglycerides (fat components in foods). Meanwhile, the antimicrobial defenses in saliva kill off some potentially harmful microorganisms before they can go any further into the digestive tract.

When you've got a bit of food, called a *bolus*, ready to swallow, it moves into your *oropharynx* (the back of your throat), ready to go down one of two side-by-side passageways. The stakes are high: If it goes down one passageway, the food successfully reaches the digestive tract and goes on to nourish you. If it goes down the other passageway, your airway closes off and you choke. You can thank your trusty *epiglottis* (a flap of cartilage) for its lifesaving feat every time you swallow, because it descends to close off your airway and your nasal passages and direct your food safely down the esophagus.

Esophagus

The next important location in the journey through the digestive tract is the *esophagus*, a long tube connecting the back of the throat to the stomach. Gravity is not enough by itself to move the food through this tube in a timely fashion, so muscular contractions called *peristalsis* automatically help push the food downward.

At the bottom of the esophagus is a ring of muscle, called the *lower esophageal sphincter*, that closes tightly after food has reached the stomach. This muscle helps keep the food and acid in the stomach from leaking backward into the esophagus.

Stomach

The next stop for food in the digestive tract is the *stomach*. Here, substances linger a while — two to four hours on average, with fats sitting longest in the stomach prior to emptying, followed by proteins and carbohydrates.

When empty, the stomach looks like a long, skinny, deflated balloon (except it's made of muscle tissue, not latex). However, the stomach can expand up to 20 times its size when needed. The average human stomach holds about 1.5 liters of food.

The stomach contains acid and enzymes to continue breaking down carbohydrates and to begin the chemical digestion of proteins. The stomach also contracts in a rhythmic fashion to mechanically mix and break down food.

A very small amount of absorption occurs in the stomach, too. Substances such as aspirin, alcohol, caffeine, and certain vitamins are directly absorbed into the body through the walls of the stomach.

Small intestine

The *small intestine* — which, if named more descriptively, would be called the very long and twisty intestine — is the next location of note in the digestive tract tour. (To be fair, the small intestine does have a smaller diameter than the large intestine. But its total length is a whopping 13 to 20 feet, or 4 to 6 meters.) There are three distinct parts of the small intestine:

>> **Duodenum:** The beginning part, immediately below the stomach. This is the most dynamic part of the small intestine, where acidity from the stomach is neutralized and the food substances are mixed with enzymes and bile that are sent in from other areas.

>> **Jejunum:** The middle part, where the majority of the nutrients are absorbed.

>> **Ileum:** The lower part, connected to the start of the large intestine, where nutrient and water absorption continues.

The interior wall of the small intestine is lined with a fine carpet of *microvilli* (tiny, hairlike protrusions), which create a huge surface area for absorbing nutrients. In total, the small intestine's surface area is approximately the size of half a badminton court. The mucus layer that forms part of the gut barrier (see the sidebar "What's in and what's out? The gut barrier decides") is also thinner throughout the length of the small intestine than in the large intestine, allowing for better nutrient absorption, including water absorption. Overall, the small intestine takes care of absorbing more than 90 percent of the fats, proteins, absorbable sugars, and fat-soluble micronutrients from your food.

WHAT'S IN AND WHAT'S OUT? THE GUT BARRIER DECIDES

The gut barrier is the master controller of which substances pass from the digestive tract into the rest of the body. This wall, which separates your gut *lumen* (or interior space) from the rest of your body, has two main components:

- **Epithelial cells:** These cells are like thin shingles that form the outer layer of your digestive tract wall, a layer just one cell thick. Between these cells are a complex network of connectors, one example being the tight junctions that hold the neighboring cells together. They form a barrier that opens and closes selectively to let things in or out.

- **Mucins:** Forming a squishy jelly on top of the epithelial cells is the mucus layer, made up of *mucins* (gel-like proteins). This mucus layer protects the epithelial cells, separating them from digestive juices, bacteria, and toxins, and helps keep the chemical environment of the lumen stable.

Meanwhile, just outside the gut barrier, various types of immune cells keep watch over the lumen to sense changes and protect against any harmful substances that may happen to get past the epithelial cell layer.

Intestinal permeability is the extent to which the digestive tract wall allows substances to pass through the gut barrier and into the body. Some intestinal permeability is needed for letting in nutrients, of course. But when your gut barrier isn't working well, in some cases it allows components of bacteria or other unwanted substances known as *antigens* to reach blood circulation and potentially cause harm. Increased intestinal permeability, commonly called "leaky gut," is associated with many chronic diseases, including inflammatory bowel disease (IBD). However, researchers emphasize that intestinal permeability is not a diagnosis in itself — it's more accurately characterized as a common underlying mechanism of various diseases.

Large intestine

The final important landscape of the digestive tract is the *large intestine*, also known as the colon. In total, it's about 3 to 4 feet long. The parts of the large intestine are as follows:

>> **Cecum:** A small rounded pouch, located where the small and large intestines meet, which aids in the absorption of water and salts.

>> **Ascending colon:** The first part of the colon. The ascending colon extends upward on the right-hand side of the abdomen.

>> **Transverse colon:** The middle part of the colon, which extends across the body horizontally, from right to left.

>> **Descending colon:** The part of the colon that extends downward on the left-hand side of the abdomen.

>> **Sigmoid colon:** The part of the colon that consists of a short, S-shaped structure that connects the descending colon to the rectum.

>> **Rectum:** A short vertical tube of muscle at the end of the colon, which holds stool before it exits the body.

>> **Anus:** The opening, controlled by muscles, through which stool leaves the body.

Unlike the small intestine, the large intestine doesn't have specialized functions within the different parts. Primarily your large intestine absorbs extra water and prepares stool to leave the body. But other crucial digestive functions occur here as well:

» Vitamins and essential minerals are synthesized and absorbed by the microorganisms living in your colon (see the section "Getting to know the microorganisms that call your gut home").

» These microorganisms also transform undigested and nondigestible components of your diet into various substances. For example, some fibers from your diet are turned into SCFAs, which supply energy to the colon's cells and also get shipped throughout the body to perform health-supporting functions.

» The gut microorganisms produce or transform several other molecules crucial for digestion and gut health: for example, they convert primary bile acids to secondary bile acids, which are needed for fat digestion.

Next, the fecal material passes into the rectum, ready to be eliminated. When the time comes for the stool to exit, it passes through your anus (which is, incidentally, much more than the butt of jokes about the seventh planet in the solar system). The anus is an opening surrounded by strong muscles, with the inner layer of muscle controlled involuntarily and the outer layer voluntarily. Both of the muscle layers relax at the moment you decide to pass stool. The journey of your food components through the digestive tract is thereby complete.

Uncovering the enteric nervous system

When most people refer to the human nervous system, they mean the central nervous system (CNS), consisting of the brain and spinal cord. But the gut is wired up with its own nervous system, called the *enteric nervous system* (ENS). The ENS is one of the three branches of the autonomic nervous system, alongside the parasympathetic division (controlling the functions of resting and digesting) and the sympathetic division (controlling fight-or-flight).

The ENS forms a network of nerves running through the walls of the digestive tract from esophagus to anus, and it's sometimes known as the "second brain." The main features of the ENS are as follows:

» The ENS contains approximately 400 million to 600 million *neurons* (nerve cells that send messages via electricity), compared with around 86 billion in the brain.

>> The ENS is made up of different types of interwoven neurons. Some of these neurons sense movement or chemicals, and others trigger action from muscles, blood vessels, mucosal glands, intestinal cells, or other structures.

>> ENS activity happens automatically and without your awareness.

The ENS is the main system responsible for keeping the harmony in your digestive tract under normal circumstances, because it coordinates both digestive and defensive functions. Specifically, the ENS does the following:

>> Controls gastrointestinal motility by regulating muscle contractions

>> Helps manage the absorption of nutrients and balance of electrolytes

>> Influences production of digestive enzymes, hormones, and mucus

>> Controls local blood flow in the gut

>> Influences gut barrier function by regulating the proteins that maintain the connections between epithelial cells

>> Shapes the production and function of immune cells to control gut inflammation

TECHNICAL
STUFF

The ENS is very sensitive and responsive because good digestion depends on it knowing what occurs at precise times and places in the gut. However, the neurons of the ENS don't reach all the way to the gut barrier, so they need to rely on intermediaries to learn what's happening inside the gut lumen. The neurons rely on signals from special cells in the epithelial cell layer, called *enteroendocrine cells*, that are attuned to changes in chemical content inside the digestive tract. When the cells are triggered, they pop out hormones of different types. (Read more about the enteroendocrine cells in the section "Grasping how hormones help your gut function.")

The ENS communicates with the CNS in various ways, but mainly through interactions with the vagus nerve, which is part of the parasympathetic (rest-and-digest) nervous system. You can find more details on the mechanisms of ENS-CNS communication in the section "Figuring Out How the Gut and the Brain Communicate."

Getting to know the microorganisms that call your gut home

The community of microorganisms that live in the digestive tract is another factor that's critical for healthy digestion and maintaining a stable gut environment.

Scientists have known for several centuries that a community of *microorganisms* (living things that are too tiny to be seen without a microscope) live and thrive in the human digestive tract. But only in the past two decades, with advances in gene sequencing technologies, were scientists able to understand the full range of microbes living there and what they're genetically equipped to do.

These microorganisms (also called *microbes*) are a collection of several different types:

>> **Bacteria:** Microorganisms consisting of a single cell, which reproduce independently

>> **Archaea:** Early-evolving single-celled microorganisms that are similar to bacteria but have a different cell wall structure

>> **Fungi:** Microorganisms made up of one or more cells, which reproduce independently through spores

>> **Viruses:** Nonliving microbes that latch themselves onto living cells in order to reproduce

The community of microorganisms living together at one site in the gut is called the *microbiota*. In everyday language, the words *microbiota* and *microbiome* are used interchangeably, but the term *microbiome* is technically much broader and encompasses both the microorganisms and their habitat, in a little microenvironment.

No two people have the same collection of microorganisms in their digestive tracts, but some overall patterns exist at each digestive tract site:

>> **Oral cavity and esophagus:** The microorganisms here are constantly changing as new ones arrive from the outside environment (mainly through ingestion of food and drink). Many of the microbes are killed off by the antimicrobial substances in saliva, but certain types make their home on your tongue and teeth.

>> **Stomach:** Under normal circumstances, the stomach (which is highly acidic) is considered a relatively sterile environment with few microbes that call it home. However, in various diseases or with exposure to acid-lowering treatments, certain microbes may proliferate.

>> **Small intestine:** A modest population of fast-growing microorganisms exists in this location. Not a lot is known about this microbial community because of the difficulty accessing this site in the body, but new technologies such as ingestible sampling devices are increasing researchers' knowledge about small intestinal microbes.

>> **Large intestine:** The large intestine is home to a massive and relatively stable community of microorganisms. Most people have between 180 and 1,000 different species of microbes represented in their large intestine, with an estimated 37 trillion to 38 trillion bacterial cells in total (in addition to other types of microbes).

Functioning together, these microorganisms in the digestive tract carry out crucial jobs for maintaining gut health:

>> **Transforming foods:** Different types of microbes in your intestines have the potential to be mini-factories, churning out molecules called *metabolites* that can act locally or be shipped around the body, fitting into the appropriate receptors like keys into locks. One example of metabolite production is when bacteria in the gut create SCFAs from nondigestible dietary fibers.

>> **Modifying medicines:** Gut microbes transform certain medicines that reach your gut, potentially either increasing or decreasing their therapeutic effects. One example is levodopa, a common medicine for Parkinson's disease, which becomes less effective when broken down by gut microbes.

>> **Helping control overall metabolism:** Microbes in your gut influence overall parameters of your metabolism (for instance, your blood sugar regulation).

>> **Keeping your immune system under control:** Gut microbes influence the development and functioning of various immune cells. They create signals to limit inflammation and keep the peace in your digestive tract.

>> **Making vitamins:** Colonic microbes are tasked with the critical function of creating vitamin K, as well as some B vitamins, which are absorbed directly from the colon.

The effects of the gut microbes clearly go far beyond digestion. Even though a germ-free human has never existed, scientists have now amassed enough scientific evidence to say with certainty that you'd have no hope of survival without your digestive tract microbes enabling key activities within your body.

Uncovering how your immune system shapes digestion and gut health

Digestion and defense are the two primary jobs that your gut must manage constantly, without taking a single day off. Defense is important because your gut can't be a free-for-all where any old substance (especially a microorganism with the potential to harm you) is welcomed into your body and permitted to circulate in your blood. Thus, your *immune system* (the network of organs, tissues, cells, and chemicals that help your body know whether to accept or reject the substances it encounters) is a very active player in maintaining harmony in your gut. Your immune system must react appropriately to every new substance it encounters in the gut: tolerating things that will benefit you (such as nutrients), and getting rid of things that may harm you (such as sickness-causing strains of *Salmonella* bacteria).

One section of the small intestine, called the gut-associated lymphoid tissue (GALT), has an especially high concentration of immune cells. However, immune interactions occur all along the length of the digestive tract. Here are the main ways the immune system participates in gut homeostasis and well-functioning digestion:

>> Immune cells interact with the gut's resident microorganisms. Certain immune cells learn to tolerate the harmless microorganisms, and in turn the microorganisms keep the immune cells from going wild and causing excessive inflammation.

>> Microbes such as bacteria can trigger the immune system by binding to special sensors on immune cells. When the sensors recognize certain markers on the microbes, a chain reaction is set off inside the immune cell, causing it to release different signals called *cytokines.* The type of microbe and the immune cell involved determine which cytokines are released, helping the body respond to infection or inflammation.

>> Immune cells called *macrophages* help maintain the integrity of the ENS. For example, they rapidly clear out debris when enteric neurons die.

Grasping how hormones help your gut function

Yet another factor necessary for smooth gut functioning is the production of *hormones* (chemical messengers) that facilitate digestion and overall metabolism. This hormone production occurs through your enteroendocrine system.

A special type of cell in the epithelial cell layer, called an *enteroendocrine cell,* is the key to gut hormone production. These specialist cells are scattered all along the gut wall, and together they make up the largest endocrine organ in the body.

Enteroendocrine cells release various chemicals in response to mechanical and chemical triggers in the lumen of the gut (such as stretching movements, nutrients, or toxins). Scientists have identified more than 20 types of hormones that can be released from these cells, including the following:

- » Cholecystokinin (CCK)
- » Corticotropin-releasing factor (CRF)
- » Gastrin
- » Ghrelin
- » Glucagon-like peptide 1 (GLP-1)
- » Glucagon-like peptide 2 (GLP-2)
- » Histamine (a compound that acts like a hormone)
- » Leptin
- » Secretin
- » Serotonin (also known as 5-HT)

Some of these chemicals act as neurotransmitters. However, the gut–produced version of these chemicals may not reach the brain or may have different effects in the gut compared to in the brain. Nevertheless, these substances are important for smooth gut functioning.

When these hormones are released, they can affect digestion by triggering the secretion of digestive juices, by activating ENS neurons directly, or by circulating in the blood and signaling faraway sites in the gastrointestinal tract or the brain.

MOTILITY: MOVING RIGHT ALONG

Motility is the movement of food and fluids (and waste) through your digestive tract. One way to measure gut motility is via *gut transit time* (how long it takes for an item of food to go all the way through your digestive tract after ingestion). The average gut transit time is around 20 to 30 hours, with anywhere between 14 and 59 hours being considered normal. Abnormally fast gut transit times can be associated with looser, more watery stools (because the stool material travels through the colon too fast for all the water to be absorbed), while slower gut transit times are associated with harder stools.

Figuring Out How the Gut and the Brain Communicate

This chapter makes clear that the normal functioning of the gut involves more than meets the eye: not just food physically moving through the GI tract, but complex coordination of the enteric nervous system as well as gut microorganisms, immune cells, and hormones that all make digestion proceed without a hitch.

But what happens in the gut definitely doesn't stay in the gut. The gut and the brain constantly share each other's business, messaging each other back and forth all day long. The channels for relaying these two-way messages between the gastrointestinal tract and the brain are called the *gut-brain axis* (or the *brain-gut axis*).

Signaling via the gut-brain axis is crucial for integrating activities between the brain and the gut, and in particular for maintaining a stable gut environment.

Here are the main channels of two-way communication between the gut and the brain (you can find more detail in this chapter's sections on brain-gut and gut-brain communication):

>> **Nerve activation:** The neurons of the ENS interact with the *vagus nerve* (part of the parasympathetic nervous system, controlling rest and digestive functions). This nerve is the main superhighway for messages between the gut and the brain. The vagus nerve can be activated either directly or indirectly (for example, by signals from gut microbes).

>> **Immune signals:** Immune cells from the gut can release cytokines and other signals that reach the brain.

>> **Hormone signals and metabolites:** Gut-produced hormones can activate ENS neurons that convey messages to the brain. Alternatively, certain hormones produced in the gut can circulate in the blood and reach targets in the brain (such as the area postrema, dorsal vagal complex, and hypothalamus). Some metabolites produced in the gut, such as SCFAs, circulate in the blood and either influence brain regions or directly reach the brain.

Messages from brain to gut

The brain communicates with every single part of your body. But in particular, the constant messages directed downward from brain to gut are crucial for maintaining good gut function, helping control everything from ENS activation to hormone production, microbiota composition, and immune activity.

Some messages that travel from the brain to the gut are the outputs of certain brain networks (in other words, multiple areas of the brain that work together to carry out a function). Important brain networks for determining gut function are:

>> **The medial prefrontal cortex (PFC) network:** This network gathers information from elsewhere in the brain and orchestrates the body and behavioral responses to stress, including the regulation of emotions.

>> **The lateral PFC and orbitofrontal cortex network:** This network integrates information on the state of the gut from multiple places, putting together a picture of food intake and visceral pain.

The output of these (and other) relevant brain networks feed into two main subcortical structures, the hypothalamus and the amygdala. They also reach the hippocampus, which handles key functions in learning and memory. From these relay stations, the information feeds down into the gastrointestinal tract and influences various aspects of gut functioning, including gut motility and your experiences of visceral pain. The brain messages and their effects occur without your conscious awareness.

Stress can have a major impact on the messages that go from brain to gut. When you experience stress (that is, mental worry or tension triggered by a difficult circumstance), a body system called the *hypothalamic-pituitary-adrenal* (HPA) *axis* kicks into action to help you manage your mental and physical responses. Even though the HPA axis helps you weather the stressful situation, its activation can temporarily disrupt some aspects of your gut functioning by increasing intestinal permeability, changing ENS neuron activity, or altering your immune system. Recent research also showed that stress can set off a biochemical cascade that changes the gut microbiome and negatively affects the intestines. When you're stressed out, the immediate effect is that brain signals may increase gut motility and secretion, causing temporary but potentially urgent gut symptoms.

In addition to these normal functions of the brain-to-gut messaging, sometimes in "emergency" situations (such as shock, severe environmental stressors, or intense fear) the HPA axis makes brain messages override gut functioning. Just as you have emotion-related facial expressions, you may have emotion-related gut patterns of movement and secretion that become automatically activated. Scientists believe these emotion-related signatures in your gut may then feed back to the CNS, telling your brain that the emotion is still being experienced. This phenomenon may prolong the effect of many emotional states on the gut even when the initiating event is long past.

Messages from gut to brain

The gut is very communicative: It gives a detailed play-by-play of everything happening in the digestive tract environment, including information about stretch and pressure, nutrients, hormones, and immune cells. And the brain keeps tabs on all of it.

What does the brain do with all this information from the gut? It integrates the data into brain networks to alter your anxiety levels and your mood. Furthermore, evidence from animals shows that some inputs from the gut may even influence the formation of memories, as well as cognitive performance and emotion-related behaviors. Very few of these signals to the brain are consciously perceived, however. Only the ultimate messages such as "I'm hungry" or "I have to go to the bathroom," which require you to act a certain way, may reach your awareness.

Messages from gut to brain can be sent in multiple ways:

» Enteroendocrine cells in the gut produce different types of signaling molecules; for example, CCK and GLP-1 can signal fullness, and ghrelin can signal hunger. Meanwhile, some signaling molecules from immune cells can convey pain, discomfort, nausea, or fatigue to the brain.

» Gut microbes can convey information to the brain that shapes how you behave, especially in response to stressful situations.

» Metabolites such as SCFAs produced by gut microbes help regulate certain brain functions and manage neuroinflammation.

Diet is sometimes an important contributing factor to these gut-to-brain messages. The ENS and endocrine system carry messages to your brain about the nutrients in your gut. A part of the brain called the *anterior insula* (aINS) receives information about the sensory aspects of your food, while the *orbitofrontal cortex* (OFC) integrates information about the food's flavor and reward value, as well as the context of food intake (such as visual and auditory signals) to influence your overall sensory perception of the food and how satisfying you find it.

Understanding How Gut-Brain Axis Signaling Differs in IBS

Given that IBS is classified as a disorder of gut-brain interaction (DGBI; see Chapter 2), it may not be surprising that gut-brain signaling in IBS doesn't happen in a typical fashion. In fact, aberrant gut-brain signaling is really the core feature of IBS. No abnormalities occur in the structure of the gastrointestinal tract, but disruptions are seen in the gut-brain axis messaging described in this chapter, leading to overlapping gut and brain symptoms.

The take-home message is that the brain plays a big part in triggering and maintaining IBS symptoms. When you have IBS, the brain is a little too good at taking the sensory input from the gut and conveying it to certain brain centers, which influences your conscious experience of abdominal pain, discomfort, and anxiety and affects your brain activity. All of this can manifest as undesired IBS symptoms. Importantly, these crossed wires in the gut-brain axis mean you may not be able to control symptoms 100 percent by micromanaging your lifestyle and everything you eat. Mind-body interventions, which engage the brain-gut axis, are needed to truly address the core deficit of IBS. (You can find out more about these interventions in Chapter 11.)

Here are some of the differences relevant to the gut-brain axis that scientists have observed in people with IBS:

>> Different patterns of brain activation in response to stimuli in the gut that are not usually painful to people without IBS, as well as different responses to painful stimuli (with more activation of emotional brain networks)

>> An increase in the size of the amygdala and/or limbic system

>> Altered ENS function, with ENS neurons sending stronger pain signals to the brain and normal gut activities such as peristalsis and gas formation being perceived as discomfort or pain

>> Abnormal operation of the HPA axis, leading to an exaggerated stress response by the body

>> Differences in the colonic gut microbial community (reduced diversity and different proportions of specific bacterial groups)

>> Increased intestinal permeability, especially in IBS-D (diarrhea)

Scientists aren't yet sure if these differences are the cause or the effect of IBS, but nevertheless they demonstrate that gut-brain axis signaling in IBS is, indeed, abnormal. Ultimately, these IBS-linked abnormalities in gut-brain communication may result in the following:

>> Chronic abdominal pain

>> Altered bowel habits

>> Ties between emotions and gut symptoms

>> Behaviors such as excessive dietary restriction, hypervigilance, or anxiety, which aren't helpful ways of managing symptoms

SENSITIVE NERVES

Some people with IBS are known to have *nerve sensitization* — in other words, the normal sensory and pain messages traveling from gut to brain through the ENS are triggered by stimuli that are normally insignificant, and may leave a memory of pain even when the stimulus is no longer present. Pain sensations can be protective and help the body avoid harmful stimuli, but they stop being protective when they're constantly triggered. Scientists have found that nerve sensitization involves some of the following changes in the brain:

- Abnormal integration of sensory input from different sites in the digestive tract and the rest of the body

- Altered balance between brain processes that stimulate pain and those that inhibit pain

- Increased neuronal firing and connections in the brain

- Reduced transmission of certain neurochemicals

Researchers have developed ways to measure nerve sensitization through different levels of mechanical, electrical, thermal, or chemical stimulation in different gut segments, with or without viewing the affected gut region. However, nerve sensitization is not usually measured in clinical practice. Mind-body interventions and other IBS interventions can reduce nerve sensitization and thereby decrease perceptions of pain.

Therapeutically addressing brain-gut and gut-brain signaling in IBS can significantly improve how you feel. (You can find out more in Part 3.)

Faulty messages from the brain

For people with IBS, the abnormalities in gut-brain communication can shape experiences and symptoms on a day-to-day basis, with the brain often triggering initial symptoms. The brain may prompt the release of various hormones that affect gut motility and the experience of pain, so you may notice the symptoms come on if you experience fear, anger, stress, or hypervigilance. Stress, in fact, is a very common trigger of IBS symptoms.

For some people, based on having a history of stress or trauma, the body may involuntarily respond to a day-to-day stressor in a more exaggerated way than normal. The amygdala in the brain controls activation of the HPA axis, increasing or decreasing the stress response. The amygdala, which generally regulates negative emotions, is also very responsive to stressors in early life, and forms links between pain experiences and emotions that may be lasting. In IBS, the amygdala is a key site that determines the effects of stress on your gastrointestinal tract. Involvement of this brain region may account for why some people with a history of traumatic childhood experiences develop IBS. Increased amygdala function is not desirable, but the good news is that amygdala function can be altered through specific brain-focused interventions (see Chapter 11).

Dysfunctional communication from the gut

For someone with IBS, the gut may sometimes instigate the cycle of brain-gut hyperreactivity. You may eat a specific food (or any food at all, really) or experience a sensation in the gut that somehow alters your gut secretions or motility.

The brain automatically perceives this change as discomfort or pain. Potentially the pain sensation triggers feelings of stress, making you change your mood or behavior. Or the pain can trigger strong emotional reactions.

A vicious cycle

The initial trigger for IBS symptoms may be a moment of stress, or it may be something you ate or drank. Whatever the initial cause, when you have IBS, the gut and the brain may continue to send SOS messages back and forth, leading to hypervigilance and perceived pain. Even after a minor disturbance, the oversensitive gut tells the brain it's experiencing pain, making the brain panic about the situation, and making the gut even more sensitive. And on and on in a continuous cycle.

Because of this vicious cycle, gut symptoms may persist in IBS even when the source of stress is removed. In Chapter 3, Michael is an example of someone who experienced a stressful period at work, triggering IBS symptoms. Yet the symptoms remained even after work became less stressful. The cycle of brain-gut oversensitivity was already initiated and proved difficult to break.

This phenomenon also explains why gut symptoms may emerge even when nothing physical has changed in the gut: The changes in chemical or neural signaling patterns are not visible or identifiable with the usual medical tests. A change in your emotional state or mood (or sometimes just thinking about eating or drinking) can bring on the symptoms, and this situation can make you worry about what to eat because it may make the symptoms worse. The unhelpful cycle continues.

REMEMBER

Yet the cycle can definitely be interrupted if you have the right tools. Part 3 goes over the different treatment options for IBS, and Chapter 11 specifically covers mind-body therapies that can be surprisingly effective and simple to implement.

2

Navigating an IBS Diagnosis

Understand the process of seeking an IBS diagnosis and what tests may be needed to rule out other conditions.

Empower yourself to stay positive and proactive with an IBS diagnosis by finding the right supports.

Chapter 5

Determining Whether You Have IBS

The current popularity of irritable bowel syndrome (IBS) has some real upsides — namely, that more and more people are empowered to talk about their gut issues. In 2006, the model and media personality Tyra Banks revealed on *The Tyra Banks Show* that she had IBS, saying she was "very gassy" and followed a low–FODMAP diet to help control symptoms. Actress Kirsten Dunst has also spoken about her IBS and its direct connection to her depression and anxiety. Social media influencers post video dispatches from the bathroom, reporting on their IBS symptoms after consuming the latest popular iced coffee flavor. This kind of sharing may help people with IBS feel less alone and make them much more open to talking about their symptoms with medical professionals and others.

TECHNICAL STUFF

FODMAP stands for *fermentable oligosaccharides, disaccharides, monosaccharides, and polyols.* Read more about a low–FODMAP diet in Chapter 8.

But one downside of all the attention and the normalization of gut issues is that IBS sometimes becomes a catchall term for digestive issues with unknown origins. Plus, it can cause some people to get complacent — some people with abdominal pain that's associated with their bowel movements are happy to go around saying, "Oh, yeah, I have IBS" without further medical investigation.

So, don't let all the IBS talk mislead you into thinking you can just apply the IBS label to yourself and get on with your life. A medical diagnosis of IBS is a crucial part of understanding your symptoms and knowing the best (and quickest) way to resolve them.

If you think you may have IBS, consulting your doctor to seek a diagnosis is critically important because:

>> Several serious conditions such as colon cancer or inflammatory bowel disease (IBD) overlap with the symptoms of IBS. Without a correct diagnosis, you may be delaying treatment for one of these conditions and putting your health at risk.

>> Studies show that if you delay an IBS diagnosis, you're more likely to develop symptoms of anxiety or depression. Or if you already have anxiety or depression, it may get significantly worse.

>> Confirming that you have IBS allows you access to the latest treatment approaches that are shown to work, beyond what you could've researched on your own.

In addition, some people who delay an IBS diagnosis may be tempted to experiment with a treatment — perhaps something they learned about on social media or a five-step plan from a diet book. But you can further complicate the situation and even harm your health if you try a treatment such as a dietary change without receiving a diagnosis first. (See the section "Watching Out When You Seek a Diagnosis," later in this chapter.)

Diagnosis is an essential first step in taking charge of your IBS. Seeking out a timely, correct diagnosis is a worthy aim, because it can open up a whole new world of options for your health.

This chapter covers what to expect when you set out to discover whether you really have IBS. It goes through the steps you need to take, including what other conditions may need to be ruled out before an IBS diagnosis can be made with certainty. The chapter also covers some of the pitfalls to watch for during the process of diagnosis.

OVERCOMING THE REASONS NOT TO SEEK A DIAGNOSIS

For people who suspect they have IBS but who don't yet have a diagnosis, many obstacles can get in the way of seeking a proper diagnosis. Sometimes a person's symptoms seem so normal that it may not have even occurred to them to consult a medical professional.

One example is Xi Chen, an internal medicine doctor at NYU Langone Health, who wrote in *Aeon* online magazine about having gut health issues during his medical school days: "I had for years suffered from debilitating GI issues that had sometimes even impaired my ability to attend classes, out of fear of having an accident on my commute. And yet, I had never thought to see a doctor about it." Chen reported that even when he became aware that the symptoms may be concerning, he tended to downplay them, feeling that he didn't want to be a burden to anyone. He wrote, "I believed that my issues were not urgent, that they were the product of fixed environmental factors, and . . . that my symptoms were simply a rite of passage into the club of normal adulthood in the modern US."

Stories like Chen's may not be unusual. But medical practitioners exist to help you decode your symptoms and guide you toward treatments that may bring relief. No doctor is going to knock on your door and ask if you have any diagnosis-related needs at the moment — it's up to you to reach out and make an appointment to discuss your symptoms. You deserve to understand your symptoms and feel the best you can feel.

Seeking a Diagnosis

For some diseases, your doctor may recommend you undergo a test (or series of tests) to help confirm your diagnosis. But for some other medical diagnoses, no single test currently exists to tell you with certainty that you have it. IBS is in the latter category. Thus, IBS diagnosis follows two basic steps:

1. Seeing whether your medical history and symptoms fit the IBS diagnostic criteria

2. Ruling out other conditions that could account for the symptoms

Historically, IBS was called a *diagnosis of exclusion* because other conditions were expected to be definitively ruled out (in other words, excluded) through a series of tests before a diagnosis was made. However, to avoid placing an undue burden of testing on people when exploring an IBS diagnosis, and because clinical diagnosis with minimal other testing tends to be accurate, it's now more common for a doctor to make a diagnosis based on the symptoms plus some simple tests to screen for other conditions. From there, additional tests may be recommended based on your personal history and initial test results. At the end of this process, a diagnosis of IBS by a qualified medical practitioner is a highly accurate classification that can unlock a variety of treatment options (see Part 3) that you may not have previously considered.

Chances are, you'll need to visit your primary care physician multiple times before you receive an IBS diagnosis. But the effort can really pay off, ultimately giving you more certainty about what accounts for your symptoms and how to move forward.

TIP

To seek a diagnosis, the first thing to do is make an appointment with your primary care provider. Your doctor may ask about your history and current symptoms and order some initial tests. Depending on the results, you may have to undergo further testing. Occasionally, you'll receive a referral to a gastroenterologist or another specialist, who will gather additional information and potentially rule out other conditions. An alternative healthcare provider such as a naturopath cannot diagnose IBS, but they may help support treatment (see Chapter 6).

Also note that when you're being assessed for IBS, you may be advised to avoid certain medications: nonsteroidal anti-inflammatory drugs (NSAIDs), like aspirin, ibuprofen (Advil), or naproxen (Aleve). These drugs can sometimes worsen abdominal pain in people with IBS, interfering with diagnosis. If you're taking these medications regularly, however, continue taking them unless your doctor recommends otherwise.

ADVOCATING FOR YOURSELF

In an ideal world, every doctor would be up to date on the latest thinking around disorders of gut-brain interaction (DGBIs) and listen carefully and empathetically when you describe your symptoms. But the experiences of people with IBS tell a different story. The majority of doctors are great listeners — they may have received training on how to be compassionate with every patient — but many people share stories online of how a doctor seemed to doubt their sincerity or downplay their symptoms. (A negative story is far more likely to be posted online than a run-of-the-mill positive experience, unfortunately.) Despite these stories, it's still important to avoid giving up on the diagnostic process altogether and self-diagnosing. An IBS diagnosis will go more smoothly for everyone if you maintain a good relationship with your doctor, and for this reason you may have to advocate for your needs calmly and kindly.

Here are some proactive tips for making sure you're properly heard during the process of diagnosis:

- Clearly state your objective at the beginning of the appointment, within the first minute if possible. For example, "I have abdominal pain every day, and I'd like to know if I have IBS."

- Come prepared with a written list of your symptoms that you can refer to (or give to the doctor). See the section "Communicating your symptoms" for tips on how to create this list.

- Make sure you mention specific examples of when your symptoms prevent you from doing what you want to do. For example, "While doing a 20-minute exercise routine last week, I had to stop twice to use the bathroom."

- Throughout the appointment, don't be afraid to jot down notes so you can review and absorb everything later. And during the appointment, try to make sure you understand what you hear and clarify if needed. You may say, for instance, "I hear you saying that stress could be the reason for these symptoms." Bringing a support person with you can be valuable as another pair of ears.

- If you arrive with specific questions, ask them at the beginning of the appointment to make sure there's time to address them. If you need to ask questions along the way, use a calm and nonconfrontational tone. For example, "If the symptoms don't go away after graduation, what action should I take?" Be aware that your symptoms may not completely go away, even if you follow all the recommended treatment options.

Remember: Respect and empathy go both ways. If the doctor has thoughtfully listened to your concerns, consider carefully what they have to say even if it's not exactly what you want to hear. Often the doctor can get all the required information from your medical history combined with a few simple diagnostic tests, so remember that asking for more tests beyond what's recommended may not be helpful and may even introduce risk and complications. After the doctor has all the information, be prepared to accept the IBS diagnosis and move forward with appropriate treatments.

Waiting for your diagnosis

If you see your doctor the same week your abdominal pain starts, you're experiencing acute pain that's not indicative of IBS. But don't hesitate to seek care if you think you should. See your doctor especially if the pain is persistent, severe, or associated with vomiting, blood in the bowels, or fever — this could prompt investigations to rule out other conditions. Be aware that although an IBS diagnosis may be suspected early, the diagnosis will only be confirmed if the pain (associated with abnormal bowel movements) persists for six months or more.

While you're waiting, be sure to document your symptoms (see the section "Communicating your symptoms") so you're prepared to provide accurate information and move forward more rapidly when it's time to dig into a diagnosis.

Assembling your medical history

Your *medical history* is information about the health of you and your biological family members in the past. The medical history is one critical step in the process of diagnosis. To obtain this information, the doctor may ask you to complete a form (on paper or online) and/or ask you questions in person.

As part of your medical history, be sure to share the following information:

>> Whether you have any previously diagnosed conditions

>> What medications you're currently taking; what supplements, vitamins, and minerals are a part of your routine; and any other substances such as alcohol or cannabis products you regularly consume

>> What surgeries and hospitalizations you've had in the past

>> Whether you've had any sudden or serious gut infections that involved vomiting and diarrhea in the past two to three years

You may also be asked for an overview of illnesses affecting the members of your immediate biological family, if known.

Communicating your symptoms

Your job when seeking a diagnosis is to document and communicate your symptoms as clearly as possible so the doctor is working with accurate information throughout the process. Your doctor may guide you through some questions to figure out the relevant details of your symptoms.

A written record is the best way to keep track of your symptoms in the days and weeks before your doctor's appointment. We list the main relevant symptoms in Chapter 2. You can create a record of symptoms for several days or a week. You can also jot down the answers to these overall questions:

>> How long has the symptom been occurring?

>> How often do you experience the symptom?

>> Is the symptom's severity always the same, or does it become milder or more intense?

» What seems to make the symptom better or worse?

» Was there a time when the pattern of your symptom seemed to change?

If you have the feeling that your symptoms are related to what (or when) you eat, keeping a one-week food diary is also a good idea. A food diary lists everything you eat, day by day. (Chapter 7 has more information on keeping a food diary.)

After you've written everything down, take the information to your doctor's appointment so you can refer back to it. You may even want to prepare a copy in case the doctor wants to keep it as baseline information, which may help track your progress over time.

Tracking your symptoms using this kind of list for at least one week before your doctor's appointment may provide useful information in the process of diagnosis. The severity of each symptom can be informally rated on a scale of one to ten, with one being very mild and ten being the worst you've ever experienced.

Undergoing tests

IBS diagnosis involves various tests that your doctor may recommend to complement the information obtained about your personal symptoms and medical history.

In addition to a physical examination, the doctor may order tests; some of the typical tests your doctor may request are listed in the following sections.

Blood tests

Various blood tests may be ordered when you're undergoing evaluation for IBS. The *anti-tissue transglutaminase (anti-tTG) test* is a blood test that helps diagnose celiac disease in people who regularly eat gluten. The anti-tTG test checks for blood levels of antibodies or immunoglobulins, which are proteins produced by the immune system in people with celiac disease.

A *complete blood count* (CBC) provides information about the cells in your blood, and is a measure of overall health as well as a way to screen for conditions such as infection, anemia, or blood disorders (including leukemia).

An *electrolyte panel* measures the levels of your body's important electrolytes (essential substances in your blood, which indicate homeostasis or balance), namely:

» Bicarbonate

» Calcium

>> Chloride

>> Magnesium

>> Phosphate

>> Potassium

>> Sodium

Altered levels of these electrolytes may occur when you have excessive diarrhea or vomiting, or disorders of the kidney or heart.

A *liver enzyme* blood test measures different substances made by your liver, and screens for liver disease or damage.

An *albumin* test measures albumin, a protein made by your liver. Abnormal levels can give information about nutritional health or signal a liver or kidney disorder.

A *c-reactive protein* (CRP) test measures your blood level of CRP, a marker of inflammation. Elevated CRP can signal the need to investigate other conditions.

A *thyroid-stimulating hormone* (TSH) test screens how well your thyroid is working. If levels of this hormone are too high or too low, it could signal a thyroid disorder.

Cross-sectional imaging

The main type of cross-sectional imaging used to rule out diagnoses besides IBS is *abdominal ultrasound.* This painless type of test uses a small device pressed against the skin of your abdomen. The device sends sound waves that are used to create an image of the structures under the skin. This test may be useful for identifying liver, bile duct, gallbladder, bowel blockage, ovarian, or uterine problems. If pancreatic problems are a concern, other tests such as a computed tomography (CT) scan of the abdomen may be more sensitive.

Stool tests

Stool tests can screen for other causes for your digestive symptoms. First, they can identify infectious microorganisms that may be present, especially when IBS-D is suspected. A *stool calprotectin test* measures inflammation in your colon and helps diagnose IBD. It detects levels of *calprotectin*, a protein that signals gut inflammation.

Endoscopic evaluations

This type of test, often done under sedation, uses a scope (tube) with a camera, which is inserted into a part of your digestive tract to view the tissues. Instruments inserted through the tube can remove growths or take tissue samples. *Upper endoscopy* focuses on your esophagus, stomach, and the first part of your small intestine (the duodenum) to diagnose conditions such as peptic ulcer disease, celiac disease, or upper GI cancer. *Lower endoscopy*, normally a *colonoscopy*, focuses on your colon. This test helps diagnose colorectal cancer, IBD, and many other conditions. One or both types of endoscopic evaluation may be required, depending on what the doctor suspects may be going on.

Breath tests

For a lactulose, glucose, or hydrogen breath test, you consume a sugar that's poorly absorbed by your body. When you have an overgrowth of bacteria in your small intestine, these resident bacteria break down the sugar and produce higher levels of the relevant gases. These gases are measured through your exhaled breath for a diagnosis of small intestinal bacterial overgrowth. This test has fallen out of favor with many medical professionals, but some medical centers may offer one of these breath test options.

Putting the pieces together

After the doctor collects all the information and test results, their next step is to integrate all the pieces and determine the most appropriate diagnostic category for your symptoms. The doctor will synthesize the evidence within your personal context, drawing on their clinical experience. This process may result in an official diagnosis of IBS.

REMEMBER

Receiving a diagnosis of IBS is a milestone in your health journey, not the end of the road. The journey toward better health continues as you delve into the various treatments that have been tested and shown to work for people with IBS symptoms like yours.

And what if, after all the pieces are put together, you don't qualify for an IBS diagnosis or any diagnosis at all? This is what happened to the author Kristina many years ago when she had occasional debilitating abdominal pain and other digestive symptoms. At first, she felt lost and discouraged by not receiving the diagnosis because she was left without any clear options for treatment. But what she has learned since, after a long process of improving her health, is that even without a diagnosis, the gut health journey continues. While she muddled through the various options for addressing her symptoms, her work as a science writer allowed her to interview many scientists on the cutting edge of the field. Years later, she's (mostly) symptom-free and ended up creating the resource she wished she'd had during her journey toward wellness: *Gut Health For Dummies* (John Wiley & Sons). The book can serve as a touchstone for anyone who doesn't receive an IBS diagnosis and wants to continue feeling empowered to improve their gut health.

Considering Other Conditions

A proper IBS diagnosis isn't complete until you've screened for, or ruled out, a number of other related conditions that can cause IBS-like symptoms. This section covers the conditions and symptoms that commonly overlap with IBS and what tests may help diagnose them. To be clear, multiple invasive tests may not be required; your doctor may diagnose IBS by confirming the symptoms along with your medical history, and screening out other conditions via blood tests and possibly ultrasound. Additional investigations may be requested as needed, personalized to your health details.

Celiac disease

Celiac disease (CD) happens when *gluten* (a protein in wheat and some other grains) triggers an immune reaction that damages the inner lining of the small intestine, interfering with the body's ability to absorb nutrients properly.

The majority of the time, CD is confirmed with an anti-tTG blood test. As long as you're currently consuming gluten, this test is remarkably accurate. However, up to 5 percent of people may have a false negative on this test. If there's continued concern that CD may be present, upper endoscopy with biopsies obtained from the duodenum is the gold standard test to confirm the diagnosis.

CD can be easily mistaken for IBS, as shown in a 2013 study that found people with CD were much more likely than others to have received a previous diagnosis of IBS, especially in the year before they received their correct CD diagnosis.

Colorectal cancer

Colorectal cancer (CRC) occurs in the colon (large intestine) and may spread to other parts of the body. According to the World Health Organization, CRC is the third most common cancer globally, accounting for one in ten cancer cases. Its seriousness should not be underestimated — it's the second leading cause of cancer-related deaths in North America.

JANE'S CASE: HIDDEN CELIAC DISEASE

Jane, a 35-year-old woman, visited her doctor with symptoms of abdominal cramping and bloating that had occurred on and off for the past five years. She reported three small, loose bowel movements per day, with no blood in her stool. She was unaware of any gastrointestinal illnesses in her family history and had assumed for the past few years that her symptoms were probably attributable to IBS. In one of her doctor's visits, Joan mentioned some involuntary weight loss over the past year, with a rash that tended to appear on the backs of her arms and upper chest. These symptoms prompted the doctor to request some blood tests, which revealed that her iron levels were abnormally low. Jane received a referral to a gastroenterologist, who suspected celiac disease rather than IBS. Accordingly, she underwent an endoscopy of her small intestine in conjunction with the anti-tTG blood test. The results both pointed toward celiac disease. Jane went on a strict gluten-free diet, and all of her symptoms resolved within six weeks.

In the past, CRC was much more likely to occur in individuals over the age of 50, but CRC rates in younger individuals have increased sharply in recent years, for reasons not yet clear (but likely driven by environmental exposures, including diet). A family history of CRC is one sign that the possibility of CRC needs to be explored.

Colonoscopy is the gold standard for the diagnosis of CRC, and noninvasive stool tests such as the fecal immunochemical test (FIT) to identify hidden blood in the stool are relatively effective for CRC screening. Regular screening (either via stool test or colonoscopy) is recommended for every person 45 and over in the United States and 50 and over in Canada, or for younger people who have a family history of CRC.

In terms of symptoms, CRC may be differentiated from IBS by the presence of unexplained weight loss, blood mixed in with the stool, or rectal bleeding, none of which normally occur in IBS. Unfortunately, CRC occurs frequently even without these alarm symptoms though, and a full medical history can provide important clues.

Endometriosis

Endometriosis is a condition in which tissue similar to the lining of the uterus grows outside of the uterus, causing chronic pain in the pelvic area, digestive symptoms, heavy menstrual bleeding, and sometimes infertility. Irregular menstrual periods are a hallmark of this condition, in addition to abdominal pain that is worst at the time of the monthly cycle.

If your doctor suspects endometriosis, referral to an obstetrics-gynecology specialist is required to make the diagnosis. IBS symptoms can be difficult to distinguish from endometriosis because, although the abdominal pain in IBS doesn't always stick to the pattern of the monthly cycle, sometimes IBS symptoms can be more severe during a person's monthly cycle.

Inflammatory bowel disease

IBD is a group of conditions that involve long-term inflammation of the digestive tract, which can be detected through various tests. IBD normally begins between the ages of 20 and 40 years, but also commonly occurs after age 60. IBD can often be managed with medications (either biologics or immunosuppressants), but no cure exists. Digestive symptoms and inflammation may go into remission with treatment and then come back when a *flare* (a sudden increase in symptoms for a period of time) occurs.

The main types of IBD that may be explored before confirming an IBS diagnosis are:

>> **Crohn's disease:** In Crohn's disease, patches of inflamed, damaged tissue can show up in different locations, with each patch extending deep into the digestive tract wall. These patches can occur anywhere along the digestive tract, from the mouth to the anus (or as it's known informally, "from gum to bum").

>> **Ulcerative colitis:** In ulcerative colitis, inflammation is restricted to the large intestine. The damage may be anywhere along the length of the colon, and it occurs only on the surface layer of the intestinal wall.

Making a diagnosis of IBD is complex and requires multiple tests. If IBD is suspected, the next steps may include blood tests, followed by colonoscopy, and then imaging of the small intestine. This imaging may include computed tomography (CT) or magnetic resonance (MR) enterography, or bowel ultrasound if available. Sometimes, these tests are insufficient, and specialized endoscopic tests of the small intestine are needed.

IBD and IBS frequently have the same outward symptoms. A 2014 study found that 10 percent of people with IBD had received a prior incorrect diagnosis of IBS. And even more confusingly, up to 35 percent of people diagnosed with IBD can have symptoms of IBS, even when their condition is in remission; this is referred to as *IBD with IBS overlay,* and it affects as many as one-third of people with IBD.

Small intestinal bacterial overgrowth

Small intestinal bacterial overgrowth (SIBO) is a proliferation of bacteria in your small intestine, which may cause symptoms such as gas, bloating and distension, diarrhea, or abdominal pain. SIBO tends to have symptoms in common with IBS-D. SIBO usually seems to arise from diabetes (which is associated with poor intestinal motility) or disorders of motility, although research continues on this topic.

SIBO is sometimes diagnosed through a breath test (measuring hydrogen, glucose, or lactulose), although these tests may have a high rate of false positive results. Your doctor may recommend a course of antibiotic treatment to address the bacterial overgrowth if SIBO is suspected; a marked improvement in symptoms could indicate that SIBO was indeed contributing to them.

Thyroid disorders

Thyroid disorders prevent your thyroid from producing the correct quantity of hormones. Too much thyroid hormone is called *hyperthyroidism,* and too little is called *hypothyroidism.* Both of these disorders are diagnosed based on information from a physical exam, medical history, and blood tests.

Additional body-wide symptoms such as tremors, sweating, or irregular heartbeat may help distinguish a thyroid disorder from IBS. But if you have IBS-like digestive symptoms, both hypothyroidism and hyperthyroidism may need to be ruled out.

Watching Out When You Seek a Diagnosis

For some people, seeking a diagnosis can seem drawn out and confusing, but patience pays off. Taking action on interventions too soon can interfere with receiving a timely and correct diagnosis.

Unnecessary surgery

Sometimes when a person has IBS, they jump to conclusions about what may be causing their abdominal pain or other symptoms, thinking that surgery will give them instant relief. Yet surgery is sometimes unnecessary, introducing extra health risks as well as costs (see the sidebar "Miranda's case: Seeking surgery").

Studies show, in fact, that people with IBS are three times more likely to have a gallbladder removed and two times more likely to have an appendix or uterus removed, only to find no improvements in their symptoms after the surgery.

For best results, follow the recommendations of the surgical specialist. If surgery is recommended, make sure you fully understand the motivation and the probable outcome after the surgery.

MIRANDA'S CASE: SEEKING SURGERY

Miranda was a 47-year-old woman, slightly overweight, who had been experiencing symptoms of alternating constipation and diarrhea for close to 20 years, associated with abdominal pain that was most noticeable on the right side, and also general abdominal cramping a few times per week. Her bowel pattern was a hard bowel movement every two to three days, which continued for up to two weeks, and then diarrhea two to three times per day for the subsequent four days. Her abdominal pain and cramping improved temporarily after passage of gas or bowel movements.

Miranda was concerned about gallstones contributing to her symptoms, and she had an ultrasound that identified fat in the liver, but no stones or abnormalities of the gallbladder. Her abdominal pain was limiting her activities and quality of life. She modified her diet on her own — cutting out lactose and carbonated drinks — after seeing some content on social media. Her diarrhea mildly improved, but her pain and constipation continued.

She requested a referral to a surgeon, because she was convinced her pain was from a gallbladder problem. The surgeon recommended a few more tests, none of which identified a problem with her gallbladder, and did not recommend surgery. Miranda was disappointed with this decision and sought the opinion of another surgeon. The other surgeon agreed surgery was not a good option, but Miranda was undeterred. Because of her progressive pain and lack of diagnosis, the surgeon finally agreed to gallbladder surgery because the symptoms were somewhat compatible with gallbladder problems. One year after gallbladder surgery, Miranda continued to have recurring abdominal pain, abdominal cramping, and constipation, consistent with IBS. All the symptoms she experienced before the surgery were unchanged.

Premature dietary changes

Even before receiving an IBS diagnosis, you may be tempted to start eliminating certain foods from your diet to see whether you get relief from your symptoms. Yet two potential problems can arise when you implement dietary changes prematurely:

>> **Cutting wheat from your diet can cause a false negative result on the blood test for CD, ruling it out when you actually have the condition.** CD is a serious condition, so you could be damaging your health if you delay a diagnosis.

>> **Following a strict elimination diet, where you eliminate several categories of food at once, can make your diet less well-rounded and in some cases put you at risk for nutritional deficiencies.**

REMEMBER

Following healthy diet guidelines (such as MyPlate in the United States; see www.myplate.gov) and making simple diet changes, such as reducing your intake of ultra-processed foods with many additives, fast foods, and sugar-containing beverages, will not impact your IBS diagnosis. Let your doctor know if you've made modest dietary changes that seem to have made a difference to your symptoms. If you suspect you may be lactose intolerant, for example, you may consider cutting out dairy products for a short time and noting whether you see a change in your symptoms.

Food intolerances can be difficult to distinguish from IBS. However, after your IBS diagnosis, you can tackle some dietary changes in a systematic way as part of your treatment approach. We detail diet-focused treatments for IBS in Chapters 7 and 8.

TIP

The upshot, however, is that you should make sure to ask your doctor before implementing any kind of drastic dietary change prior to seeking an IBS diagnosis.

Possible Future Diagnostics for IBS

Although there's no single diagnostic test for IBS right now, many researchers around the world are on a quest to find one. Various kinds of tests have been proposed for identifying IBS over the years, but so far no test has stacked up as a reliable way to diagnose the condition. This section covers some promising tests you may hear about that are not currently useful for diagnosing IBS.

Blood tests

One potential test, already on the market, is a blood test based on antibodies to gut-nerve-damaging toxins that are produced by some bacteria such as *Salmonella*. The test accurately identifies the anti–cytolethal distending toxin B (anti-CdtB) and anti-vinculin antibodies, but further validation of the test is needed because not all people with IBS may actually have high levels of these antibodies. So far, nothing from this test would be likely to change your approach to managing IBS, so doctors don't typically recommend it.

Gut microbiota tests

Tests of the community of microorganisms living in the gut have been proposed as a way to diagnose IBS. Although gut microbial tests are available to purchase by mail order, the results are not standardized and they currently provide no information relevant to an IBS diagnosis. Taking such a test is not recommended. In the future, scientists may determine the features of the gut microbiota that are relevant to IBS diagnosis, and at that time, a medical-quality and clinically useful test may be developed.

Chapter 6

Moving Forward with an IBS Diagnosis

After you're diagnosed with irritable bowel syndrome (IBS), a unique emotional journey may begin as you shift into a new way of understanding your health. Each person may react to an IBS diagnosis in a slightly different way, and all reactions are valid — from relief to confusion to anger and everything in between. Here are some examples of how people have reported feeling after receiving an IBS diagnosis:

» Shannon felt a sense of relief because, with a family history of colon cancer, she had been worried that her symptoms indicated a tumor.

» Barbara felt uncertain and overwhelmed because, even though she knew she would need to change her diet patterns after her IBS diagnosis, she didn't know where to begin.

» Amir felt dissatisfied and skeptical when he received the IBS diagnosis because he had been certain his symptoms were general digestive issues that would someday disappear once and for all.

» Isabella felt angry about her IBS diagnosis, thinking how unfair it was that she had to deal with the condition for the rest of her life when she used to go anywhere and eat anything she wanted.

Others report having so many thoughts and emotions after an IBS diagnosis that they can't identify a single one that's dominant — and that's valid, too. Whatever you think and feel after you receive an IBS diagnosis, your immediate job is to take a breath, feel those feelings, and let all the thoughts come and go from your mind. Your role is to be a silent observer of these emotions and thoughts. Simply being aware of how IBS is affecting you can help you with acceptance while reducing its control over your life.

This chapter is an opportunity to zoom out from your day-to-day experiences and see yourself from a bird's-eye view as someone who may have a variety of thoughts and emotions about your diagnosis of IBS. It's a chance to consciously adjust your mindset to set you up for positive action and create a map of people who can help and support you through this journey. With this approach, you'll be able to accept your diagnosis and take charge of what you think and feel, ending up stronger and more capable than ever.

Coming to Terms with Your Diagnosis

Receiving an IBS diagnosis (see Chapter 5) is a critical first step in taking control of your health. Being diagnosed is a significant milestone because it moves you from someone who experiences gut symptoms of mysterious origin to someone with a specific, named disorder. This gives you the IBS keyword that's helpful not only for online searches, but also for connecting with others who have closely related experiences. From a medical perspective, the IBS descriptor also links your condition with the thousands of research studies conducted by scientists and doctors over the years, unlocking knowledge about what may treat your symptoms effectively.

A number of simple actions, such as naming your emotions, gaining more information, and committing to care for yourself can help you accept the diagnosis as well as your feelings about it, and help you move forward in a positive and proactive way.

Naming your emotions

Initially, a diagnosis of IBS can spur various emotions — which don't always diminish as time goes by. Sometimes during your health journey, you'll be struck with a feeling of sadness or frustration for no apparent reason. But emotions don't need to be justified — they happen when they happen.

TIP

The healthiest way to handle emotions is to acknowledge them and express them in appropriate ways while not letting them dictate your overall behavior. During the turmoil of negative emotion, the simple act of naming the emotion can reduce its power over you. If you're experiencing negative emotions, try to take a step back and identify what you're feeling. If you keep a record of symptoms (see Chapter 5), you can write the feeling down under the notes for that day. These simple acts can help you keep the bigger picture in mind, remembering that emotions come and go naturally (see the sidebar "Learning to surf the waves").

Gaining more information

One of the best things you can do to help you understand and embrace your IBS diagnosis is to get up to speed on the latest medical information about the disorder. Reliable, up-to-date information can be incredibly empowering. And guess what? Gaining such information is exactly what you're doing by reading this book. Bravo!

TIP

Reading this book, however, should be only part of what you do to learn about IBS. Many other great sources of information exist. Here are some tips on finding high-quality information about IBS:

>> If you find information online, check the source and try to see whether it's been verified by a medical professional or other reputable person. Don't rely on help generated by artificial intelligence (AI), like ChatGPT, Gemini, or Meta AI — it can be inaccurate.

>> When choosing books to read, check the credentials of the authors. Look for medical professionals experienced in IBS treatment who aren't trying to simultaneously sell you an IBS solution.

>> Be cautious of the information about IBS you find on social media. Whether or not the person is a medical expert, they often gain more attention by saying something surprising than by saying something true.

Sometimes gaining more knowledge and a deeper understanding of what you're experiencing can help you feel more in control of your IBS, even without exploring new treatments. For example, Chapter 4 explains the biological basis of gut-brain communication and the importance of paying attention to your mental and emotional state. And if you want to learn about different treatments, science-based information about IBS will help you find out which ones have been tested in scientific studies and shown to work across large groups of people — not just a treatment reported to work for one paid influencer.

Committing to care for yourself

When you have IBS, it's common to feel like you're always playing catch-up with your symptoms, just barely coping with one symptom before you're hit unexpectedly with the next one.

TIP

You'll be in a much stronger position to deal with your IBS if you make a personal, internal commitment to take charge of giving your body the care it needs, whether or not you have symptoms at that moment. This commitment means taking on the responsibility of full-time caregiver to your body, being open and adaptable to providing what it needs. Your commitment will almost certainly require some lifestyle adjustments (see Chapter 12).

Staying positive about your IBS diagnosis

All feelings, both positive and negative, are valid during your IBS journey. But it's important not to let negative emotions become a barrier to seeking help or moving forward in your life. If left unmanaged, negative emotions can lead to unhelpful behaviors such as a general lack of activity and social contact, which can worsen your health overall. Thus, you may need to employ strategies for acting positively and in your best interests as a person with IBS.

Staying positive doesn't mean seeing the bright side of every situation (spoiler alert: diarrhea doesn't always have a bright side). Nor does it mean denying the emotions you experience, such as sadness and anxiety. It means embracing and acknowledging those emotions, and still managing to act in a positive and proactive manner that helps you control your IBS. Staying positive helps you think clearly about treatments and avoid acting out of desperation, leaving you better off in the long run.

So, how can you act in a positive way on those days when everything feels terrible? Sometimes medical professionals or other people can support you through these tough times (see "Finding Your Support Team," later in this chapter). But there are also some things that you can do to help yourself stay on a positive track when you experience the bouts of negative emotion that are normal for all people with IBS:

>> **Setting aside time for activities you enjoy for their own sake:** For example, you may enjoy sitting on a bench in the park, playing a musical instrument, or crafting.

>> **Writing down everything on paper:** Sit down with a pen and paper and write in a stream of consciousness, not paying attention to spelling or sentence flow. After you're done, you may choose to tear up the paper and discard it.

>> **Spending time with someone you trust:** Simply hanging out with a friend, a family member, or another person with IBS can be its own medicine. You may choose to share your emotions with them, or you may not, but the important thing is that you spend time with someone who leaves you feeling better off.

REMEMBER

And don't forget that IBS can bring you advantages, too. It's easy to focus on what IBS takes away, but IBS can also bring the opportunity to see the world in a different way and gain superpowers that don't come easily to IBS-free people. Here are some of the possible benefits that IBS may bring:

>> **Making you a kinder and more empathetic person:** You'll likely be more empathetic toward others who are experiencing digestive troubles or other kinds of challenges in their lives.

>> **Requiring you to be aware of behaviors that positively impact your health:** When your body gives you no choice but to maintain your healthy habits such as exercising, you have a better chance of living a longer and healthier life.

>> **Modeling important self-care behaviors to others:** You can be a great role model for your family and friends, especially for younger people.

>> **Giving you the ability to celebrate the small wins in life:** Only people with IBS know the true happiness and pride that can come from a successful bowel movement!

>> **Making you better at thinking ahead and anticipating the needs of yourself and others:** Don't be surprised if people name you as the person they'd choose to be with if stranded on a desert island!

Make no mistake: Life with IBS won't always be a picnic. But when put into perspective, you can have a positive mindset overall and even find benefits from your experiences with IBS. Just as you extend kindness and empathy to yourself in your daily life, you can spread kindness and empathy to others and make the world a better place.

Staying in the moment

With IBS (and life in general, for that matter), you only ever have to deal with the moment in which you're currently living. The past has already happened and can't be changed, while the future hasn't happened yet and can't be predicted. So, focusing on living in the moment is one of the best skills you can develop to help you live a fulfilling life. Living in the moment is a day-to-day practice of regularly quieting the thoughts running through your mind and really focusing on what you're experiencing through your five senses: what you see, hear, smell, taste, and feel.

Try it now if you can: Wherever you are, inhale a long, slow breath that lasts around 10 seconds. Feel the breath draw in and reach every part of your body. Then let it out just as slowly, letting all your thoughts drain away from your mind. Then breathe slowly and normally and start to notice all the details around you, including what colors and shapes you see, and all the little sounds you hear. Notice how your clothing feels against your skin and the temperature of the space. As you continue to breathe, notice how the different parts of your body are feeling.

This exercise may take less than a minute overall, but it's one example of how powerful it can be to quiet your mind and pause the cycle of worry and anticipation about your next IBS symptom. To help you develop the practice of living in the moment, many wellness practitioners offer video tutorials, books, and courses. When practiced regularly, this technique may lead to a more positive mindset and increased freedom from negative emotions.

Finding Your Support Team

In a June 2024 episode of the game show *Jeopardy!*, the host, Ken Jennings, got to the part of the show where he asked contestants to share some information about themselves. A contestant from Seattle called Hakme Lee shared how she decided her husband was a keeper in the early stages of their relationship. She said, "I have IBS, which is medical speak for I go to the bathroom when I'm nervous. I was very open about that with him. On our third date, which was dinner at his place, I go to his apartment, he takes my coat, and then he guides me by the elbow and shows me where the bathroom is." Jennings reacted with a smile, saying, "What's the opposite of a red flag? I love that."

Information about your health is yours to decide whether to share — so you definitely don't have to disclose you have IBS on national television. Nor do you have to share about your IBS with friends or family, unless you want to (see the sidebar "Creating your IBS elevator pitch"). But many people with IBS feel secure and supported when they talk to selected people about their IBS and develop a network of people they can open up to. Studies show, in fact, that when people with IBS feel they have a social support network, they report experiencing less pain. That's right, social interactions actually modify the structure and function of the pain networks in the brain.

As the person with IBS, you're the one who decides which people qualify as members of your IBS support team. This section goes over some of the types of people who you may decide to bring into that trusted circle. Some of the qualities of a good support person are:

>> Accepting your IBS rather than denying the condition or its impacts

>> Validating your feelings rather than brushing them aside

>> Honoring any request to keep the information you share confidential

>> Listening when you talk about the hard experiences (within a reasonable time limit) and not trying to give unsolicited advice

>> Helping you brainstorm or problem-solve when you specifically ask for advice

Everyone with IBS deserves understanding and support. Your list of cheerleaders may look different from that of another person with IBS — but the important thing is that a few people know the basics of your condition and can support you in various ways.

Primary care physician

A primary care physician (sometimes called a general practitioner or family doctor) is a healthcare professional who gets to know you over time and understands the big picture of your health. This doctor may be the one who diagnoses you with IBS. Although the primary care physician may not be able to explain everything about IBS in a few short appointments (after all, this 300+ page book just barely covers it), but they may be able to support you by:

>> Coordinating testing and referring you to the appropriate specialists to address specific symptoms

>> Providing treatment options

>> Connecting you with other healthcare professionals, such as registered dietitians, or to support groups

Remember to communicate clearly and calmly with your primary care physician (see Chapter 5) about how IBS is affecting your life and what problems are a priority for you to solve.

Specialist physicians

Specialist physicians include gastroenterologists, psychiatrists, internists, or others who address specific areas of medical specialty. Although you may not be able to see a specialist as frequently as you see a primary care physician, they may have access to more solutions in their specialty area. Professional associations may be able to help you find specialists who frequently treat IBS.

A specialist physician may be able to:

>> Address specific symptoms or ways that symptoms affect you, sometimes providing access to new options.

>> Provide access to specific tests to secure an IBS diagnosis.

>> Help you create a personalized action plan that encompasses lifestyle solutions and prescription medications.

>> Give you advice about less frequently used medical strategies that are not included in usual IBS clinical guidelines.

Your appointment with a specialist may not be very long, so make sure you come prepared and clearly communicate what you're hoping to address. Writing down your most pressing questions in advance of your appointment is advisable to help you clarify your thoughts.

Registered dietitian

A registered dietitian has a science degree that focuses on nutrition. In many countries, dietitian is a protected title that indicates a professional is accountable to a regulatory body for high standards of education and ethics.

Many people with IBS (although not all) benefit from dietary changes as part of their IBS treatment plan. A registered dietitian can be an incredibly helpful member of your care team. They can

>> **Answer questions about diet and IBS.** A dietitian can provide clear answers to your questions about how food affects IBS and overall wellness.

>> **Clarify food myths.** With so much inaccurate content found online and on social media, a registered dietitian can address and debunk common misconceptions about food and its impact on your health.

>> **Provide nutritional education.** A dietitian can let you know the best practices to enhance and maintain your health through diet at different life stages.

>> **Help you figure out if you're a good candidate for addressing your IBS symptoms by altering your diet.** The low-FODMAP diet or another dietary intervention works well for many people with IBS, but a dietitian can help determine whether you're likely to benefit from dietary changes.

>> **Assist in identifying food triggers.** When you want to change your diet to improve your IBS symptoms, a dietitian can help you navigate the process of discovering and managing your specific food triggers.

>> **Help set dietary goals.** They can help you set personalized goals for symptom management that align with your unique needs.

>> **Offer meal and recipe suggestions.** Dietitians can recommend meals and recipes tailored to your preferences and dietary needs, or even help develop a customized diet plan that ensures you meet all your nutritional requirements.

TIP

To get the most out of your appointment with a registered dietitian:

>> **Reflect on your goals.** Consider your objectives for the visit and what you hope to walk away with — whether it's a whole new dietary plan or adjustments to your current diet.

>> **Maintain a food and symptoms diary.** Track your food intake and symptoms for at least three days.

>> **Prepare your questions.** Bring a list of questions or concerns you'd like to address during the visit.

>> **Bring a medication and supplement list.** Bring a comprehensive list of all medications and supplements you're currently taking.

A dietitian may be available through your healthcare plan or for private consultation, either online or in person.

Other medical professionals

Other medical professionals may be helpful as members of your support team:

>> A **psychologist, gastropsychologist,** or **counselor** to help you deal with the emotional and interpersonal aspects of living with IBS.

>> A **social worker** to help you access resources such as community services, financial assistance, and employment supports.

Alternative healthcare practitioners

Around half of people with IBS end up seeking support from a practitioner of alternative healthcare (sometimes called *complementary and alternative medicine,* or CAM) outside of the mainstream medical system. Some of the common practitioners that help people with IBS are

>> Acupuncturists

>> Ayurvedic practitioners

>> Kinesiologists

>> Massage therapists

>> Naturopaths

>> Traditional Chinese medicine practitioners

Sometimes conflicting recommendations may arise between medical professionals and alternative healthcare professionals. The treatments offered by CAM practitioners may not have scientific evidence showing that they work broadly for people with IBS, but these highly personalized treatments may bring relief of some symptoms.

REMEMBER

Generally, for a chronic condition such as IBS, having more treatment options to choose from is a good thing, particularly if you've explored a range of possible treatments with your medical team and you still have symptoms. Just be mindful of the budget you set for these treatments, because some CAM treatments can end up being very costly with minimal benefits.

Household members

If you live with others, chances are, your household members know about some of the ways you care for yourself with IBS, whether it's spending extra time in the bathroom or accommodating a special diet. Your household members can support you in various ways:

>> **Offering practical help:** When you're not feeling well, your family or house-mates may be able to pick up the slack by assisting with chores, running errands, or driving you to appointments.

>> **Giving you space:** Sometimes the thing you need is alone time to deal with your symptoms. With good communication, you can let your household members know when you need some space without causing conflict.

>> **Learning about IBS:** If your family or housemates learn about IBS, they may be more likely to understand what you're going through and more willing to accommodate your needs in a flexible manner.

>> **Following your lead:** Your household members can pay attention to your energy levels and mood day by day, being responsive to what you need while giving you autonomy to make your own decisions around food and activities.

TIP

Sometimes bathroom schedules and special eating patterns can cause tension in a household where everyone has different needs. Then again, tension is almost inevitable from time to time when any people are living in close quarters. You can help avoid problems through good communication and planning ahead when possible. (Chapter 13 has some helpful strategies.)

Family and friends

Selected family members and friends can make great allies in your IBS journey. The choice of whether to tell someone about your IBS and seek their support is yours to make and depends on your relationship with each person. Some people may feel comfortable telling their parents or siblings, and others may feel more comfortable relying on a couple of close friends and no family members.

No matter whether your trusted family members and friends live nearby or far away, they can support you in different ways. For example:

>> Listening when you want to talk and validating your feelings

>> Accommodating your dietary needs at a get-together and checking in advance about anything that may make your visit more comfortable

>> Accompanying you to a medical appointment if you request their presence

>> Being your point person during a social function — getting you an item you need or covering with an excuse if you have to leave suddenly to deal with symptoms

TIP

Being able to rely on a trusted person can make all the difference to how you feel, but everyone has their limits around how much time and energy they can devote to supporting others. Try to expand your trusted circle to a few different people that you can seek support from at different times.

Other people with IBS

Having IBS can sometimes feel lonely — especially if you've ever had to leave a fun social gathering to lock yourself in the bathroom and deal with symptoms. But given that more than 10 percent of people worldwide have IBS, you're definitely not alone in your experiences! And other people with IBS can be an excellent source of support and ideas.

TIP

You can connect with others who live with IBS in a variety of ways:

>> Read books or blogs by people who write about their experiences living with IBS. Some organizations focused on digestive disorders have patient stories on their websites.

>> Follow people on social media who live with IBS and post publicly about their experiences.

>> Join an online group (for example, on Facebook or Reddit) where you can read and post questions.

>> Participate in a virtual event held by an organization focused on digestive disorders. Many events provide an educational talk by an expert and an opportunity to ask questions.

>> Meet up in person with other people diagnosed with IBS, perhaps as part of a support group. (If no support groups exists in your area, consider starting one yourself!)

>> Get involved in patient advocacy activities through a support organization (see the sidebar "Looking for IBS support organizations").

LOOKING FOR IBS SUPPORT ORGANIZATIONS

Many organizations around the world offer information and support for people with IBS. You can look internationally, nationally, or locally for organizations that support gastrointestinal disorders in general or IBS specifically. These organizations, even if not based in your country, often have websites that are excellent sources of information — many of them have stories from real patients and some offer IBS support groups, either online or in person. Some of them have fundraising initiatives such as charity runs that give you a chance to participate in a rewarding volunteer experience. Some examples of reputable organizations include:

- **Canadian Digestive Health Foundation:** https://cdhf.ca/en
- **GI OnDEMAND:** https://gi.org/practice-management/gi-ondemand
- **The IBS Network:** www.theibsnetwork.org
- **International Foundation for Gastrointestinal Disorders:** https://iffgd.org
- **Rome Foundation:** https://theromefoundation.org
- **Tuesday Night IBS:** www.tuesdaynightibs.com

CREATING YOUR IBS ELEVATOR PITCH

People with IBS or any other chronic condition may find it enormously helpful to create an *elevator pitch* — a short explanation (brief enough to be conveyed in an elevator ride) that you can use in almost any situation to make people aware of your needs. An elevator pitch is a way to help others understand your situation better so they're more likely to attribute your behavior to your condition ("She's not feeling well") rather than to your inherent qualities ("She's irresponsible"). Clinical and organizational psychologist Dr. Dayna Lee-Baggley recommends giving your elevator pitch to everyone you know because it can help preempt difficult situations. If you require a person's help or understanding later on, you can simply remind them of your elevator pitch rather than giving it to them for the first time. This helps you advocate for yourself and may make you feel more empowered when the unexpected happens.

(continued)

(continued)

A good elevator pitch focuses on the symptoms rather than the diagnosis and talks about specific behaviors that are relevant. For example, on the first day of a new class, you might tell the instructor, "I have a digestive condition that means I need to go to the bathroom sometimes on short notice. I'm going to sit near the back of the room, and if you see me leaving in the middle of a lecture you'll know why."

When you give the elevator pitch, you can also practice setting boundaries around the information you feel comfortable sharing. If someone asks for further details, you can say in a calm and friendly manner, "That's all I feel like sharing right now."

When some people hear the elevator pitch, they'll likely jump in with advice they believe may be helpful. You don't have to get into a conversation about the merits of their suggestions — just make a neutral comment such as "Interesting" or "Thanks, that may be worth considering" and move on to another topic.

3
Managing IBS

Discover the power of diet to manage IBS symptoms.

Pick a diet that may improve your digestive symptoms.

Understand the medications that effectively treat IBS.

Navigate the world of dietary supplements and learn which ones really work for IBS.

Realize how effective mind-body treatments can be for IBS and know your options.

Adjust your lifestyle, including sleep and stress levels, to improve your IBS symptoms.

Find tips and tricks for how to live well with IBS.

Chapter **7**

Changing Your Diet to Manage IBS

G iven that the best-known jobs of the digestive tract are to digest and absorb food, someone who's diagnosed with a gastrointestinal (GI) condition often immediately jumps to the question: "What should I be eating?"

When you have irritable bowel syndrome (IBS), scientific evidence shows that adjusting what you eat can go a long way toward reducing your symptoms. Thus, many medical experts suggest dietary change as one of the first things you should consider after you're diagnosed with IBS. Dietary change is also recommended by several professional organizations as a first-line treatment for IBS. (Note that throughout this chapter, *diet* refers to the entire list of what you eat, rather than the restrictive food pattern that some people imply when they say they're "on a diet.")

Even though diet can be a powerful way to take control of your IBS, don't expect it to solve everything. For the best outcomes in IBS, your treatment needs to take a holistic approach that encompasses the following possible components:

» Dietary changes

» Other lifestyle changes (see Chapter 12)

» Mind-body interventions (Chapter 11)

» Medications (Chapter 9)

» Possibly supplements or other interventions (Chapter 10)

This chapter helps you understand the role of diet in reducing IBS symptoms, and the pros and cons of changing what you eat. It covers the basic components of diet and the practical steps toward dietary change, from limiting certain foods to a complete dietary overhaul. (See Chapter 8 for more details on diets that improve IBS symptoms.)

Knowing the Role of Diet in IBS

As recently as the early 1990s, diet was not a mainstream medical treatment for IBS. Many doctors during that time remember being in a difficult position clinically: Despite their patients with IBS saying that diet affected their symptoms, everyone's experience was slightly different, and very little scientific evidence existed to help guide diet recommendations one way or the other. The best that medical professionals could do was recommend basic rules around eating, such as having regular mealtimes and avoiding overeating.

By the early 2000s, however, research began to emerge showing that a certain dietary pattern was remarkably effective for improving IBS symptoms. The game-changing diet was called *low-FODMAP*.

TECHNICAL
STUFF

FODMAP stands for *fermentable oligosaccharides, disaccharides, monosaccharides, and polyols*. Read more about a low-FODMAP diet in Chapter 8.

Diet research in the field has come a long way in the past two decades, and dietary changes are now considered one of the top treatment approaches for most people with IBS. A 2022 study in Belgium found that, in a head-to-head comparison, a dietary intervention worked better than a common antispasmodic medication (otilonium bromide) for reducing IBS symptoms. At this stage of the research, scientists have found several variations of diets (see Chapter 8) that successfully reduce symptoms for people with IBS. The studies have revealed the broad patterns, which need to be personalized to everyone's unique situation.

Before considering changing *what* you eat, you should consider implementing some basic strategies around *how* you eat. These surprisingly simple actions, which cost you very little time and money, may go a long way toward making your symptoms more manageable:

» Having meals at regular times

» Eating small, frequent meals and avoiding eating too little or too much at once

>> Eating mindfully, free of distractions

>> Chewing your food well

In addition, some basic diet strategies include:

>> Staying hydrated by drinking enough water

>> Reducing your intake of alcohol, caffeine, and carbonated drinks

>> Avoiding artificial sweeteners and ultra-processed foods that contain many additives

>> Limiting fatty and fried foods

The degree of change you should make in your daily diet depends on your personal situation and what you usually eat (otherwise known as your *baseline diet*). The main consequence when your diet is less than optimal is the lack of control of symptoms, or the possible development of nutrient deficiencies or unwanted weight gain or weight loss. In IBS, for example, if you avoid eating because you're afraid of symptoms occurring, you may develop more gas, bloating, or pain — creating a vicious cycle that possibly leads to long-term anxiety or fear around eating.

Whatever situation you're in, this chapter helps you understand what the science says about diet in IBS and what gives you the best chance of reducing your symptoms.

Determining the benefits of changing your diet

The primary benefit of changing your diet is improvements in your IBS symptoms. Overall, studies show that, for many people with IBS, a dietary change can help manage abdominal pain, bloating, diarrhea, and intestinal gas, and improve their quality of life.

Changing your diet, however, is not a 100 percent guarantee that you'll become symptom-free. Just when you think you've figured out the perfect diet for controlling your symptoms, your IBS may take a turn for the worse. Or sometimes you may eat one of your worst food culprits by accident and not experience any symptoms. However, adopting specific kinds of diets in IBS can go a long way toward stabilizing your digestive troubles, giving you more control and empowering you to seek out other kinds of treatments as well.

REMEMBER

If you're one of the lucky people who seem to get rid of your IBS symptoms altogether when you change your diet, don't make the mistake of thinking that your IBS was really a simple food intolerance all along. IBS is complex, and it shows up differently over time. Just because you remove one main factor that contributes to faulty gut-brain interaction doesn't mean you've removed all susceptibility to IBS symptoms. Depending on what's going on in your life, the symptoms may return even if you manage your diet perfectly. But you can rest assured that by paying careful attention to diet, you're giving yourself the best foundation for controlling your symptoms in the long run.

Considering potential drawbacks to changing your diet

Diet can be incredibly effective for improving your IBS symptoms. But sometimes changing your diet also comes with costs, which you should consider before making a major shift.

Consider how much time and money the dietary changes will cost and determine if you have the capacity for these costs. For example, depending on the nature of the dietary change, you may have to prepare more foods yourself at home or purchase specialty foods, such as lactose-free milk or gluten-free flour. You may also have other household members' needs to consider. Ask yourself whether you can realistically commit to implementing a new diet to achieve the potential payoff of reduced symptoms. (For tips, see Chapter 17.)

In addition, a dietary change that's not properly implemented can end up harming your health in several ways, which are listed in this section. Some people with IBS independently start to avoid many categories of foods or excessively limit their diets because they believe it helps them control symptoms on a day-to-day basis. But unexpected problems may arise as a consequence: nutritional deficiencies, disordered eating patterns, or weight loss or gain. Importantly, overly restrictive diets can also negatively affect your mental well-being. They often take a toll on emotional health by increasing the difficulty of enjoying meals and socializing with friends, leading to feelings of isolation and frustration. If you find yourself in this situation, seek the help of an experienced professional such as a registered dietitian to help you expand your diet in a way that supports your better health and well-being while maintaining control of your IBS symptoms.

Nutritional deficiencies

Nutritional deficiencies are reduced levels of one or more nutrients that prevent the body from being able to perform its normal functions. Such deficiencies can have serious consequences for your health, especially over the long term.

Nutritional deficiencies can arise in IBS when diet becomes overly restrictive (as when you eat only a few foods or not enough food to meet your nutritional needs), or when major food categories are removed (for example, eliminating most grains).

Here are some nutrient deficiencies sometimes seen in people with IBS:

>> **Fiber:** Because of either food avoidance or a special diet that may be low in fiber, some people with IBS don't get enough fruits, vegetables, and grains to meet their daily fiber needs. Fiber is essential for digestive health and a lack of it can lead to worse or more complicated GI symptoms, as well as fatigue. Fiber is also necessary for supporting a diverse community of gut microorganisms that helps you maintain your health over the long term.

>> **Vitamin D:** Vitamin D deficiency is common because of the limited dietary sources that contain vitamin D and the lack of consistent sunlight exposure in northern latitudes. Adequate vitamin D is essential for immune function and gut health. A 2015 study in Saudi Arabia found that 82 percent of people with IBS were deficient in vitamin D, compared with 31 percent of people without IBS.

>> **Iron:** A lack of sufficient intake of iron in the diet can lead to iron deficiency and iron-deficiency anemia. This state can result in fatigue, weakness, and other symptoms. About half of people with IBS have lower-than-normal levels of iron.

>> **Magnesium:** IBS patients, particularly those with diarrhea, may lose significant amounts of magnesium. This mineral is essential for muscle function, nerve signaling, and cardiovascular health.

>> **Calcium:** People who avoid dairy due to lactose intolerance or digestive issues may have lower calcium intake, increasing the risk of deficiency. Calcium is particularly important for bone health and muscle function.

>> **Zinc:** Diarrhea can lead to a loss of zinc, an essential mineral for immune function, skin health, and wound healing.

Maintaining a balanced diet and monitoring potential deficiencies through regular health checkups can help manage these risks in IBS patients. Depending on the exact nutritional deficiency and its severity, it may be addressed through improvements in your diet or with supplements. Consult with a health professional before taking any supplements — they can guide you toward the ones that are safe and effective for you.

Disordered eating patterns

Another risk of overly restrictive diets for IBS is that they may promote disordered eating patterns. A *disordered eating pattern* is a way of eating that departs from cultural norms (for example, restricting food during most of the day).

Not all disordered eating patterns in people with digestive issues are harmful or considered clinical eating disorders. Sometimes these behaviors are a normal way of coping with symptoms; other times they contribute to poor health. For example, a person may follow a low-FODMAP diet for four to six weeks to manage IBS symptoms, and then gradually reintroduce foods to figure out which ones cause issues. When they realize which foods cause symptoms and avoid these specific foods over the long term, it's a healthy response to their situation. However, an unhealthy pattern of disordered eating is if someone with IBS limits their diet to just ten foods they consider safe, refuses to try reintroducing other foods, and requires supplement drinks to get enough nutrition. A disordered eating pattern can have psychological effects and eventually cross the line to becoming an eating disorder.

Here are some examples of eating disorders:

>> **Anorexia:** An eating disorder characterized by food restriction and an intense fear of gaining weight, as well as a distorted way of seeing one's own body (known as *body dysmorphia*). It can cause severe weight loss and *malnutrition* (which is any version of inadequate nutrition, including when you have one or more nutritional deficiencies), as well as other serious health problems. Anorexia is relatively uncommon in people with IBS, but it's worth being aware of because of its serious health consequences.

>> **Bulimia:** An eating disorder marked by episodes of consuming atypical large amounts of food in a discrete period of time where there is a feeling of no control. After each episode the individual may try to vomit, exercise excessively, fast, or abuse laxatives.

>> **Avoidant/restrictive food intake disorder (ARFID):** A condition of severely limiting the amount or types of foods consumed, causing nutritional deficiencies or weight loss. Individuals with ARFID may lose interest in eating and avoid certain foods based on sensory characteristics, experiencing distress when confronted with foods they find unappetizing. However, those with ARFID don't necessarily have the fixation on body image that is present in people with anorexia. ARFID is a recently defined disorder that first appeared in the *Diagnostic and Statistical Manual of Mental Disorders* (DSM), which lists officially recognized mental health conditions, in 2013. According to estimates, around 20 percent of people with IBS experience ARFID. See the sidebar "Dealing with ARFID" for more information.

>> **Orthorexia:** A harmful obsession with healthy eating, which causes someone to restrict their diet and may lead to nutritional deficiencies and weight loss. Individuals with orthorexia are fixated on the quality, rather than the quantity, of what they eat, and they often spend an excessive amount of time on food research. Up to one-third of people with IBS may develop orthorexia, which is roughly double the rate in people without IBS.

REMEMBER

If you suspect you have an eating disorder, speak with a healthcare professional.

Also note that if you have an eating disorder before IBS arises, the eating disorder can be exacerbated by IBS symptoms or by your attempts to address your symptoms through dietary change. If you have a preexisting eating disorder, always work under the guidance of a registered dietitian when implementing dietary changes for IBS.

FOOD FEAR AND AVOIDANCE: A VICIOUS CYCLE

In IBS, it's normal to avoid certain foods because they trigger your symptoms. However, at some point, the avoidance and diet restrictions may become more extreme, resulting in ARFID. Registered dietitian Wendy Busse (https://wendybusse.com) developed a model called the *Conditioned Food Avoidance and Sensitivity Trap* (C-FAST) to explain the vicious cycle of dietary restriction and worsening symptoms that can occur in IBS. According to this model, when a person overly restricts their diet, they may develop fear of certain foods, which leads them to associate foods and physical sensations with danger. They therefore become conditioned to avoid foods, which increases their sensitivity to those foods. The sensitivity leads to unpleasant physical sensations, reinforcing food-associated fear.

If you recognize the C-FAST trap early, you may be able to break out of it. Wendy Busse suggests contacting a doctor or dietitian if you notice the following warning signs that you're caught in this negative cycle:

- **Constant or suspicious thoughts about food:** Thinking a lot about the potential negative consequences of eating certain foods.

- **Frequent food-related research:** If you're spending a lot of time on internet food research, it's a sign that your trust in food has deteriorated.

- **Emotional or physical tension:** If tension arises when you eat or think about food, food may be a stress trigger.

The good news is that you can help prevent this trap with some positive practices as you embark on a therapeutic diet for IBS. Remember these tips to maintain a healthy relationship with food as you navigate a restrictive diet:

- **Find professional support.** Getting help from a registered dietitian who specializes in IBS helps you maintain perspective on how food is truly impacting your symptoms.

(continued)

(continued)

- **Remember that elimination diets are experimental.** A diet that restricts certain foods is meant to be a temporary test to see how your symptoms improve. Many foods that you first eliminate may be tolerated later on (at least in small amounts).

- **Withhold judgment until the end.** Stick to the diet for the predetermined amount of time and make note of your symptoms without constantly analyzing whether your diet is helping. You're likely to have good days and bad days. Afterward, you can go through your notes and try to identify a pattern.

- **Keep living your life.** Don't let your life completely revolve around your diet. Continue to socialize and engage in meaningful activities.

- **Minimize food research.** Don't go down a rabbit hole of food research online. When you read about the possibility of foods causing digestive distress, you may have a heightened awareness, and it may become a self-fulfilling prophecy.

Difficulty maintaining a healthy weight

The unpredictability of IBS symptoms may increase the difficulty of maintaining healthy lifestyle habits. For example, people with IBS may rely on easily digestible but high-calorie foods, or they may restrict physical activity because of discomfort. These factors may result in energy intake being higher than energy expenditure, increasing the challenge of maintaining a healthy weight. Some studies have found that individuals with IBS are more likely to be in the overweight or obese category than people without IBS, increasing their risk for chronic inflammatory conditions such as type 2 diabetes, heart disease, stroke, metabolic dysfunction-associated steatotic liver disease (MASLD), and certain cancers.

To help maintain a healthy weight when implementing dietary changes for IBS, aim to consume a well-balanced whole-food diet that takes into account your dietary restrictions. A registered dietitian can be immensely helpful in achieving this goal. Pay attention to other parts of your lifestyle, too: Stay hydrated, aim for at least 30 minutes of moderate activity daily, and implement mind-body interventions to help maintain a calm mental state.

Reviewing the Diet Basics

When you open the door to changing your diet in IBS, you may encounter a barrage of information on nutrition, from FODMAPs to fiber and from trigger foods to tryptophan. It can be enough to make your head spin.

Before delving into what aspects of your diet you can change to reduce symptoms in IBS, ground yourself in the basic concepts relevant to your diet: macronutrients, micronutrients, and overall dietary pattern.

Macronutrients

No matter what diet you consume, it's made up of three main categories of foods — carbohydrates, protein, and fats — collectively called *macronutrients*. These macronutrients are the building blocks that you can assemble in different configurations to make up your overall diet. Each food has different proportions of these macronutrients. Humans need a balance of all three for optimal health, whether they have IBS or not.

The following sections offer a breakdown of the three macronutrients.

Carbohydrates

Sometimes called *carbs*, these macronutrients supply most of the body's energy in the form of sugars, starches, and fibers. A category of carbohydrate-rich foods called *refined grains* (which includes white bread, white pasta, white rice, and baked goods) are digested quickly and tend to increase your blood sugar after you eat them. Overconsumption of these refined grains may lead to obesity, diabetes, or metabolic syndrome.

On the other hand, complex carbohydrates, such as vegetables, fruits, and nuts, take longer to digest. In fact, some components can't be digested by the human body at all, so they travel down to your colon where they're finally broken down by the microorganisms that live there, thereby feeding the microbial community. Complex carbohydrates help keep your blood sugar stable and hunger under control.

Protein

This macronutrient is made up of different configurations of chemical building blocks called *amino acids*. Various types of protein help you build and repair body tissues, including those in your muscles, vital organs, bones, nails, and hair. Protein molecules are mostly digested in the stomach and small intestine, with a small proportion being digested in the colon.

Fats

Fats are energy-dense substances that your body stores for use when carbohydrates have been depleted; they're required for proper cell function. They're critical for the immune system, as well as for nutrient absorption and hormone production. Digestion of fats is a multistep process that involves different chemicals in your body acting on the fats you consume to break down those fats into smaller and smaller pieces. However, not all fats are created equal — some types of fat are considered healthier than others. For example, the fat found in avocados, nuts, and olive oil (called monounsaturated fats) and the omega-3 fats found in fatty fish such as salmon, as well as flaxseeds and walnuts, support a healthier gut. Trans fats and omega-6 fats (for example, corn, safflower, and soybean oils), which are often found in processed foods such as baked goods, cookies, and potato chips, can increase inflammation in the gut.

Micronutrients

Micronutrients are vitamins and minerals that you need to consume in small quantities to stay healthy. Essential micronutrients include all vitamins, as well as substances such as calcium, magnesium, iron, zinc, and iodine. Plant-derived molecules, called *polyphenols*, are also considered micronutrients; in the digestive tract, some of them lead to the growth of beneficial gut microorganisms.

Micronutrients are obtained through your diet or through supplements. (For vitamin D, however, you can consume it through fortified foods or your body can produce it in response to sunlight.) Unless you have a confirmed micronutrient deficiency, the preferred approach is to obtain micronutrients through a variety of whole foods rather than by supplementation.

Water

Although water is not a macronutrient or micronutrient, and it doesn't provide energy or calories, water is essential for life. Staying hydrated is key for digestive health, nutrient absorption, and even for managing stress.

Dietary pattern

Your *dietary pattern* is the types and amounts of foods you consume regularly, and the timing of when you consume them, over a long period of time. Scientists who study dietary patterns zoom out from the details of what people eat every day and focus on what they have a habit of eating over the long term.

Short-term consumption of foods doesn't determine your dietary pattern. For example, if you buy a box of summer peaches and eat three of them each day for a week, and then go back to your normal practice of eating one piece of fruit per day, the single fruit per day would be a part of your dietary pattern.

Research has established that your dietary pattern has the power to either protect your lifelong health or increase your risk for many chronic illnesses. Some examples of dietary patterns are:

>> **Western diet pattern:** This diet is characterized by a high intake of sugar- and fat-containing foods, with a low intake of fiber. Typically, a Western diet pattern includes many ultra-processed foods containing emulsifiers, artificial colors, sodium, and other additives — such as when someone eats fast food, salty snacks, and sweetened coffee drinks daily. This diet pattern is associated with obesity and heart disease, as well as other chronic diseases.

>> **Mediterranean diet pattern:** This diet consists of a variety of plant foods (fruits, vegetables, legumes, whole grains,) and healthy fats (olive oil, nuts, and seeds), as well as moderate intake of fatty fish, seafood, and poultry, with dairy, red meat, processed foods, and sweets being limited. The Mediterranean diet pattern is considered the gold standard for supporting health and lowering the risk of chronic diseases.

Implementing Dietary Changes in IBS

When you're ready to dive into dietary change for IBS, the plan often requires several different steps. Overall, your main task is usually to adapt your short-term diet to reduce symptoms, and then to figure out a long-term plan that supports your optimal nutrition. These tasks are described further in this section.

For best results throughout all these stages, work with a registered dietitian experienced in managing GI conditions, who can bring clarity to the very complex undertaking of dietary change and can help minimize the frustrating trial-and-error process.

Addressing mealtime routines and how you eat

A first step for nearly all people with IBS is to address your eating routines. Often overlooked, your typical meal habits and the manner in which you eat can be incredibly important factors in how food affects you in IBS. For example, consider a simple snack of peanut butter on a rice cake. If you're in a hurry and eating the snack while driving a car, it may well bring on your IBS symptoms. But if you eat the same snack in a calm and quiet room, free of distractions and mindfully enjoying every bite, it may not bring on any symptoms.

Consistency is key when it comes to eating well in IBS. Eating your meals at consistent times of the day can help regulate digestion and reduce symptoms such as bloating, gas, and irregular bowel movements. Regular meal patterns may also prevent overeating or extended fasting, both of which may trigger or worsen IBS symptoms.

Mindful eating involves paying full attention to the experience of eating, without distraction. This practice has numerous benefits for both mental and physical health and is particularly important for those living with digestive conditions.

Here are some of the benefits of mindful eating:

» **Improved digestion:** When you eat mindfully, you're more likely to eat at a slower pace and chew your foods more thoroughly, allowing your digestive system to process the foods more efficiently. The next time you sit down to eat, think about how many times you chew your food. A rule of thumb is to chew each mouthful 10 to 20 times before swallowing.

» **Portion control:** Mindful eating helps you tune into your body's hunger and satiety signals. Instead of eating until your plate is empty or eating out of habit or emotion, mindful eating encourages stopping when you're satisfied. This naturally leads to better portion control and can help prevent overeating. Portions matter in IBS because certain foods are tolerable in smaller amounts and intolerable in larger amounts.

» **Stress reduction:** Mindful eating brings attention to the present moment and can act as a form of meditation. Focusing on the sensory experience of eating, such as the taste and texture of food, can reduce stress and anxiety by diverting the mind away from worries or distractions and allowing you to fully experience the present moment. This relaxed state also aids digestion.

Eliminating common dietary culprits

As a next step for most people with IBS, some general changes in diet can be implemented if you haven't already done so. Some foods and beverages, which are outlined in this section, commonly cause IBS symptoms or make them worse. These items don't provide unique nutritional value, so most people with IBS benefit greatly from limiting them as much as possible.

Alcohol

Alcohol is a colorless liquid produced by sugar fermentation, and it's found in alcoholic beverages such as wine, beer, and hard liquor. Even if consumed in moderate amounts, alcohol can irritate the digestive tract, leading to heartburn, inflammation, and other GI symptoms. In some cases, it can also increase diarrhea. For best results in IBS, eliminate alcohol or limit it only to special occasions.

Caffeine

Caffeine is a stimulant that increases alertness and is found in foods such as coffee, tea, chocolate, and cola soft drinks. Caffeine stimulates the digestive system, which can lead to diarrhea or urgency in people with IBS. The effects of caffeine may be felt immediately or sometime after the food or beverage is consumed. Some individuals with IBS-C (constipation) may find coffee or other caffeinated beverages helpful for stimulating a bowel movement, but caution is warranted because caffeine can also irritate a hypersensitive gut and increase other symptoms.

TIP

You may have to experiment to see how much caffeine you can tolerate — the typical recommendation is no more than three cups per day of caffeinated coffee or tea, no matter which type of IBS you have.

Carbonated drinks

The bubbles in carbonated drinks such as cola and seltzer are made with carbon dioxide, which adds air into the digestive tract. This extra air increases pressure in the gut, potentially worsening symptoms such as gas, bloating, abdominal pain, and heartburn. Carbonated drinks, even if they're low in sugar and caffeine-free, should be limited as much as possible when you have IBS.

Fried foods

Fried foods such as french fries and fried chicken are known to slow down digestion because of their high fat content. They can make bloating, gas, and diarrhea worse, and they can also trigger heartburn. People with IBS should try to limit fried foods as much as they can. If you cook at home, try replacing deep-fried foods with a version made using an air fryer.

Spicy foods

Spicy foods such as chili peppers and hot sauce contain capsaicin, a chemical compound that can irritate the digestive tract lining in some individuals and cause abdominal pain or other symptoms. If you have IBS, try to eliminate spicy foods completely or use hot spices in moderation.

Artificial sweeteners

Artificial sweeteners, particularly from the sugar alcohol family (for example, sorbitol, mannitol, and xylitol), are poorly absorbed in the digestive tract and are among the most universal gut irritants in IBS. They can lead to increased gas, bloating, and diarrhea in some people. These ingredients, commonly found in sugar-free chewing gum and packaged foods such as protein bars, should be avoided as much as possible in IBS.

Ultra-processed foods

Ultra-processed foods typically contain many additives (preservatives, colorings, flavorings, emulsifiers, and artificial sweeteners), along with refined sugars, oils, and fats. Many of these ingredients can trigger digestive discomfort in IBS. Typically, people with IBS are better off when they focus on eating whole, fresh foods for the majority of their diet.

TRIGGER FOODS 101

A *trigger food* is something you eat that's consistently associated with one or more of your IBS symptoms and seems to be a cause of the symptom(s). Chances are, you've already made some observations about your diet vis-à-vis your symptoms and may be able to identify some specific foods that trigger them. For example, you may notice that when you eat fried foods you have more frequent bowel movements that day. Trigger foods are very individual, so a food that triggers one person's IBS symptoms may be completely fine for another person with IBS. The mechanisms behind what makes something a trigger food are complex and involve both the digestive tract and the brain.

Identifying trigger foods can be difficult because your body's reactions may seem unpredictable — what triggers symptoms one day, such as an apple with peanut butter, may not cause any issues on another day. Trigger foods can change over time, and they may depend on what else you're eating. (Read more about the reasons for this unpredictability in Chapter 8.)

For identifying trigger foods or ingredients, a food diary (see the section "Assessing suitability for a dietary change," later in this chapter) becomes invaluable for helping you solve the puzzle. A food diary allows you to track not only what you eat but also other factors that may be influencing your symptoms. For example, did you eat something earlier in the day that could've contributed to your reaction to a food later in the day? Were you eating in a rush or dealing with a stressful situation? All these factors can play a role, and a diary helps you see the full picture. (For a digital option, the Monash

University FODMAP Diet app (www.monashfodmap.com/ibs-central/i-have-ibs/get-the-app) includes a food diary.)

If your trigger foods aren't clear even after you make use of a food diary, you may be better off implementing a broad dietary shift such as the low-FODMAP diet (or another diet, as detailed in Chapter 8) and, over time, reintroducing categories of foods that don't trigger your symptoms.

ANNA'S CASE: SIMPLE DIETARY CHANGES

Anna was a 24-year-old woman who worked as a bartender and also played guitar in a band that had frequent late-night gigs. For the past several years, she had experienced diarrhea along with recurrent stomach pain. She noticed that fried foods seemed to bring on her symptoms, but no other foods seemed to be a particular trigger. After seeking help from her family doctor, she was diagnosed with IBS. Anna was then referred to a registered dietitian. When the dietitian asked about Anna's typical eating habits, Anna said she generally slept until midday, had a few cups of coffee, and then grabbed a burger or a club sandwich with extra bacon at work before clocking in for her shift. She sipped on juice or carbonated drinks while she worked. Late at night, after her bartending shift, she would usually eat a bowl of cereal at home in front of the TV.

The dietitian recommended working toward a NICE diet (see Chapter 8), which meant eating smaller and more frequent meals with limited caffeine, while reducing intake of carbonated drinks and juice and replacing them with water and herbal teas. Anna managed to switch out the coffee for a smoothie before work. She skipped her heavy prework meal and instead, at midday when she woke up, ate overnight oats or a whole-grain wrap with chicken and lettuce. She sipped from an insulated mug of peppermint tea during her bartending shifts. Within three weeks, Anna reported that the diarrhea was occurring only once every three to four days, and the stomach pain was almost gone.

Assessing suitability for a dietary change

After implementing the basics — addressing your meal routines and limiting or eliminating foods that commonly cause symptoms — it's time to look at what you currently eat and determine what kind of dietary change (if any) is the most suitable in your personal situation.

The most important tool at this stage is a food diary, which is a list of all the foods and drinks you consume over a certain time period. You can create a food diary on your own with a notebook or in the notes app on your phone: Write down the date and list everything you consume, both foods and beverages, and the time you consumed it. Be as specific as possible and list the brand names of any packaged foods, as well as the approximate portion sizes. Optionally, you can add details on your symptoms, stress levels, social activities, and anything else happening that day. Keeping a food diary for at least three days is usually a good basis for decisions when you're considering a dietary change.

Changing and personalizing your diet

After you decide which dietary pattern you want to implement with the aim of improving IBS symptoms — perhaps one of the diets described in Chapter 8 — it's time to take the plunge and try out the new eating pattern.

WARNING

A common mistake people make is not allowing enough time to fully assess whether a diet is working. Whenever you try out a new diet, sticking with it for a set period of time is crucial. Normally at least four weeks is enough time to determine whether a new dietary pattern is working for you.

As you implement a diet, it's a good idea to continue with your food diary and track your symptoms, because this will help you decide if the intervention is working. If the intervention doesn't seem to be working, a dietitian may be able to use the diary to identify potential symptom triggers that you may have overlooked. Remember that every dietary intervention should be personalized for your situation — a process that inevitably comes with some trial and error. Turn to Chapter 8 to read more about diet personalization.

Expanding your diet to meet your nutritional needs

The problem with some dietary interventions is that they successfully improve symptoms, but they may not provide you with complete and balanced nutrition. So, after you get a handle on your food triggers and successfully reduce your symptoms, you need to look at expanding your diet to meet all your nutritional needs for the long haul.

Let's say you've stuck to the low-FODMAP diet for four weeks and noticed a dramatic improvement in your symptoms. You may feel so much relief that you're tempted to adhere to the diet forever, but that's not a good idea — the low-FODMAP diet lacks fiber and may also lack important vitamins and minerals, which support your long-term health.

REMEMBER

You need to reintroduce foods and food categories back into your diet one by one, in a systematic way, to determine whether you can tolerate them. This helps you expand the variety of foods you eat and reduces the chance of any health effects from poor nutrition. You can find more details on food reintroduction in Chapter 8, in the section on the low-FODMAP diet.

THE FIBER PUZZLE

Before the low-FODMAP diet was widely studied, increasing fiber intake was a common recommendation for people with IBS, whether IBS-C or IBS-D. Yet some people with IBS experienced more symptoms when they increased fiber consumption, and other people experienced more symptoms when they decreased fiber. As time went on and researchers' understandings of IBS and the gut microbiome increased, they began to realize that different fiber sources had different effects and that a more nuanced approach was required in IBS.

Dietary fibers (found in foods such as fruits, vegetables, legumes, and whole grains) are typically classified as either soluble or insoluble:

- **Soluble:** *Soluble fibers* dissolve in water to form a gel within the gut and are easily fermented by the microbes in the digestive tract. They're found in foods such as oats, barley, legumes, the flesh of fruits and vegetables (with kiwi being popular), and seeds (for example, flaxseeds and chia seeds). Banana flakes also contain soluble fiber. Psyllium contains a special soluble fiber that forms a gel but isn't easily fermented by gut microbes, and it can be helpful for both diarrhea and constipation.

- **Insoluble:** Insoluble fibers don't dissolve in water and are not broken down by gut microbes but can be helpful if you have constipation. Whole grains such as bran, as well as vegetable skins, nuts, and seeds are good sources of insoluble fiber.

For many individuals with IBS, insoluble fibers can be difficult to tolerate, so soluble fibers are a better option. Based on scientific studies, there's no consensus on which fiber is best across the board. If you've been advised to try increasing your fiber intake, always introduce fiber gradually over several days to allow the digestive system to adjust. Start by adding a small amount beyond your normal diet and monitor any changes in your symptoms. Even if your symptoms slightly increase, you can stick to the smaller added amount for a few days and see if your body adapts. Adequate hydration goes hand in hand with fiber for best results, so drink plenty of water when you're working to increase the fiber in your diet.

Chapter **8**

Implementing a Diet That Works for You

E very person with irritable bowel syndrome (IBS) seems to have a slightly different story about the diet that works best for them. Some people find that their symptoms are reduced when they simply eliminate caffeine and carbonated drinks. Others keep their symptoms under control by reducing intake of lactose-containing foods (dairy products). Most people with IBS, however, need to go a little further for symptom relief — they need to make substantial changes to what they eat.

A growing number of scientific studies from around the world clearly show the benefits of certain diets for reducing IBS symptoms. The diet shown to work for the highest number of people with IBS involves eating only foods that are low in a group of fermentable carbohydrates called FODMAPs, an acronym standing for *fermentable oligosaccharides, disaccharides, monosaccharides and polyols. Fermentable* refers to substances that are broken down chemically by bacteria in the gut, thereby stimulating the growth or activity of these bacteria. In other words, the low-FODMAP diet is the most universal IBS-friendly diet. For many people, the diet provides a realistic way to reduce symptoms, providing a baseline of control so other treatments can be added on top.

WARNING

A note of caution, however: The low-FODMAP diet is not meant to be followed long-term because it lacks essential forms of fiber, limits food diversity, and can have negative effects on gut microbes. After the initial strict phase of elimination (lasting from four to six weeks), the goal is to reintroduce FODMAP-containing foods systematically to identify which ones cause symptoms for you personally. Because this diet is the most effective known dietary approach for IBS, the recipes in this book (Chapters 18 through 21) are all low-FODMAP and Chapter 17 gives you tips for success on this diet.

Even though the low-FODMAP diet has emerged as the most effective diet for improving IBS symptoms, several other diets (outlined in this chapter) are shown to work for some people, too. Each diet works in a slightly different manner to reduce symptoms, often involving multiple mechanisms within the body. Ultimately, however, the power of diet is that it can change motility, influence fluid and gases within the gut, and ultimately regulate stool formation, abdominal pain, and other symptoms.

This chapter delves into the details of the low-FODMAP diet and other diets that may be recommended for reducing IBS symptoms. It covers the decisions you need to make about your diet and how to implement the diet you choose. The chapter also warns about several diets that are not recommended if you have IBS.

Setting Up for a Dietary Change in IBS

Making a big shift in your diet requires preparation and commitment. If you had the goal of driving across the country, you'd need to make a plan before pulling out of your driveway. Similarly, before you make a big dietary shift, you need to make sure you've got a strategy in place to see it through to completion.

Choosing a diet

When making a big dietary change to alleviate your IBS symptoms (in contrast with simply eliminating common food culprits as outlined in Chapter 7), you first need to decide which diet is right for you.

Depending on your personal situation, you may want to consider opting for one of the evidence-based diets detailed in this chapter: the NICE diet, the low-FODMAP diet, the FODMAP gentle diet, the gluten-free diet, or the Mediterranean diet.

Here are some scenarios and the approaches to diet that may be most suitable:

>> **If your diet is already very restricted (for example, you eat less than ten types of foods or eliminate important categories of foods such as dairy products and grains),** it's important to seek out professional advice because further restrictions, such as the low-FODMAP diet, are not likely to benefit you. Non-diet treatments may be more suitable.

>> **If you're underweight or have a diagnosed eating disorder,** see a registered dietitian to help with a personalized approach that involves fewer food restrictions. A restrictive diet approach may not be the best option for you.

>> **If you don't have a lot of control over your own meals (for example, if you're a student who subscribes to a cafeteria meal plan),** you may choose the NICE diet, which can be easier to implement than some other diets and doesn't require a lot of specialty foods.

>> **If you feel overwhelmed by the list of low-FODMAP foods and aren't sure you can stick to it,** either a FODMAP gentle diet or a gluten-free diet can be easier to grasp and may achieve similar symptom reduction to low-FODMAP.

>> **If you don't like the idea of restricting foods or if your current diet is high in sugary and fatty foods,** the Mediterranean diet may be a good choice because it allows you to focus on including a diverse range of plant-based foods to support your long-term health.

Predicting in advance which diet will work best for you is difficult, but with some realistic assessment of your situation (and possibly a professional's help) you can select a diet that gives you the best chance of reducing your symptoms.

Deciding on the length of time

Many IBS-friendly diets involve constant vigilance about what you eat, and some of them restrict one or more categories of foods. Furthermore, sometimes your body takes a while to adapt to a new diet. These factors can make it hard to persist with a dietary change for long enough to see a difference. Thus, it's important to decide in advance how long you'll stick to the diet you've chosen, to give it a fair chance of reducing your symptoms. Knowing the diet is just for a set period of time may help you persist even if you don't see results right away.

Most professionals recommend sticking to your chosen IBS diet for four to six weeks. By then, the difference (or lack thereof) that the diet makes should be apparent. In some cases, however, you may be lucky enough to see improvements within a shorter period of time.

Documenting your progress

Your normal life doesn't necessarily come to a halt when you shift your diet to reduce your IBS symptoms. Many factors can affect your perception of how much your symptoms are (or aren't) improving, including your general mood and your stress levels. So, instead of relying on a vague sense of whether the diet is improving your symptoms, it's best to keep a record of your symptoms so you can look back later and compare. (You can find an example of a symptom tracking record in Chapter 5 or read how to track food and symptoms in Chapter 7.) You can also make note of other factors, such as your social activities and mental well-being, because these may help or hinder the effects of a dietary change.

Ideally, if you stick to the diet for the predetermined amount of time, your symptom diary will show improvement in your symptoms. But you also gain valuable information if your record doesn't show any improvement. If that's the case, you've given the diet a fair chance and you know it doesn't work for you, so you can move on to another approach.

REMEMBER

It may be unrealistic to expect all your symptoms to go away. What you're aiming for is an improvement in your symptoms to some degree. Your best chance at being symptom-free is to implement other treatments in addition to diet (which are outlined in Chapters 9 through 12).

Choosing a Diet to Calm Your Symptoms

Several diets, outlined in this section, are shown in scientific studies to help reduce symptoms in people with IBS.

NICE diet

The National Institute for Health and Care Excellence (NICE) is a nondepartmental public body in the United Kingdom that publishes guidelines for improving health and social care. This organization released guidelines on diet for IBS, known as the NICE diet.

The NICE diet is relatively simple to implement, so it's sometimes recommended as first-line therapy for people with IBS. Scientific studies show it may achieve almost as much symptom reduction as the low-FODMAP diet.

WHAT AFFECTS THE SUCCESS OF A DIETARY SHIFT IN IBS?

Some people with IBS report that they tried a low-FODMAP diet in the past and saw no noticeable improvements, but they tried again a few years later and saw dramatic positive changes. How can the same diet fail at first and then start to work well for the same person? Many factors contribute to the success of an IBS-focused diet at any point in time. Sometimes a better understanding of the diet means sticking more closely to the rules and being less likely to accidentally ingest problematic foods, and sometimes your lifestyle sets the stage for better success. Other times, psychological factors, such as your expectations, play a role. Biological factors such as the community of microbes in your gut may also influence your response, but these factors require much more research before they'll be useful in clinical practice. Ultimately, if one IBS-friendly diet doesn't work for you now, don't be afraid to try it again in the future when your lifestyle or situation changes.

This diet takes a holistic approach, restricting a short list of foods while also making recommendations for eating behavior. The NICE diet involves implementing these actions:

>> Drinking plenty of hydrating fluids, such as water and herbal teas

>> Limiting tea and coffee to three cups per day and reducing intake of alcohol and carbonated drinks

>> Limiting fresh fruit to three portions per day

>> Eating meals slowly

>> Eating at regular times and avoiding long gaps between meals

>> Eating reasonable portions and avoiding overeating

In addition, this diet recommends avoiding:

>> Sorbitol (a sugar alcohol)

>> *Resistant starches* (starchy carbohydrates that resist digestion in the small intestine and reach the colon intact), often found in unripe (green) bananas, cooked and cooled potatoes, rice, pasta, and cooked and cooled oats

>> Foods high in fiber (such as bran cereal and brown rice), which may cause gut irritation (so you can replace them with oat-based products)

>> Caffeine

>> Any personal food triggers

The theory behind this diet is that making some basic changes to calm the digestive tract can go a long way toward symptom relief. The diet removes the most commonly irritating foods while encouraging regular, moderate eating patterns. Many people see a response within six weeks of implementing this approach, but the response time can vary depending on the individual and the severity of their symptoms. If the NICE diet effectively reduces your symptoms, it's safe to maintain for a long period of time.

Low-FODMAP diet

The low-FODMAP diet is the all-star diet for reducing IBS symptoms, with many scientific studies showing its effectiveness. More than two-thirds of people with IBS see a significant reduction in their symptoms when they implement this diet, and it's shown to be effective for all IBS subtypes: IBS-C (constipation), IBS-D (diarrhea), and IBS-M (mixed).

The IBS symptoms that tend to be improved on a low-FODMAP diet are:

>> Bloating

>> Diarrhea

>> Flatulence

>> Overall symptoms

Certain carbohydrates are the affected macronutrient in the low-FODMAP diet. The basic idea is to omit or limit foods containing carbohydrates that are fermented (broken down) by bacteria in your colon, causing the production of gas and leading to digestive symptoms.

The types of carbohydrates that are restricted on a low-FODMAP diet are:

>> **Fermentable oligosaccharides:** The *O* in *FODMAP*, oligosaccharides are carbohydrates with molecules containing anywhere from two to ten simple sugars. The most well-known types of oligosaccharides are fructo-oligosaccharides (FOS) and galacto-oligosaccharides (GOS), which are also considered *prebiotics* (substances that feed microbes in the gut to benefit your health). Examples of foods high in FOS or GOS include black beans, garlic, leeks, onions, and raisins.

>> **Fermentable disaccharides:** The *D* in *FODMAP*, disaccharides are carbohydrate molecules that consist of two simple sugars joined together. *Lactose* (the sugar found in milk and other dairy products) is a disaccharide made up of two sugars, galactose and glucose.

>> **Fermentable monosaccharides:** The *M* in *FODMAP*, monosaccharides are simple sugars — for example, glucose, fructose, and galactose (found in honey and mango, for example). Fructose is very slowly absorbed in the small intestine, so when it's consumed in excess, it may pass into the colon, where it is fermented by microorganisms and may cause digestive symptoms. However, glucose may mitigate its poor absorption if it's present in proportion to fructose; glucose is readily absorbed and may take fructose with it.

>> **Fermentable polyols:** The *P* in *FODMAP*, polyols are sugar alcohols — in other words, sugar molecules with an alcohol group attached. Common polyols are isomalt, maltitol, mannitol, polydextrose, sorbitol, and xylitol. They're found naturally in foods such as avocado, celery, and mushrooms.

All these types of carbohydrates are either slowly absorbed or not at all absorbed in the small intestine. Studies show that when FODMAPs are consumed, they increase water in the small intestine and then move further down to the colon, where they're fermented by the gut microorganisms to produce gases. In people with IBS who may have gut hypersensitivity, this process causes uncomfortable symptoms. The low-FODMAP diet works by eliminating these categories of tough-to-digest carbohydrates.

WARNING

Most people's symptoms respond to this diet within one to two weeks, and the phase of restricting FODMAPs should last for no more than eight weeks. Following the low-FODMAP diet for longer than eight weeks is not recommended because it excludes nutrient-dense foods and many sources of dietary fiber. The long-term avoidance of these foods could lead to deficiencies in micro- and macronutrients. Not only that, but continuing with the diet can cost additional time and money and have negative effects on mental health and quality of life.

One other reason to implement the low-FODMAP diet only for a short period of time is that, despite the benefits to symptoms, research shows that this diet can negatively affect the gut microbiota. One of the key features of the low-FODMAP diet is elimination of oligosaccharides — and this category includes the prebiotics FOS and GOS, key substances that feed the microbes in your gut and benefit your health. Indeed, studies show gut microbial changes and a reduction in *bifidobacteria* (a group of health-associated bacteria) in the gut microbiota of people on a low-FODMAP diet. Thus, the restriction phase of the diet should be followed by a period where you reintroduce higher-fiber foods (potentially including prebiotics) back into your eating regimen.

The low-FODMAP diet has three phases, which are outlined in this section:

1. Restriction

2. Reintroduction

3. Personalization

These three phases are important to follow when you implement a low-FODMAP diet to ensure you don't end up with worse symptoms and inadequate nutrition. Because the restriction phase of the diet is fairly rigid, some people give up halfway through implementation. If you don't think you'll have the perseverance to stick to this diet and complete all three phases, you may consider trying the FODMAP gentle diet instead and adjusting as necessary to reduce your symptoms.

Restriction

In the first phase of the low-FODMAP diet, a specific list of foods is omitted or limited to very small amounts. The aim is to reduce overall intake of FODMAPs so your digestive tract has an easier time digesting your food. Animal-based protein in its natural forms (cooked beef, chicken, fish, and pork) and fat sources (olive oil, as well as plain vegetable and seed oils) are generally fine, but you need to limit certain carbohydrate-containing foods (namely, those with fermentable carbohydrates).

Table 8-1 is a partial list of foods to eat and avoid in the restriction phase of a low-FODMAP diet.

If you look through the list of foods to avoid and realize it includes many high-fiber foods that are generally known to support your health, you're absolutely right. The low amounts of fiber and several other critical nutrients are why it's critical for the low-FODMAP restriction phase to last no longer than eight weeks. Even though you may be thrilled to see a reduction in your symptoms, you may put your health at risk or develop a nutritional deficiency if you stick to this phase for too long. The goal is to reduce pressure on your digestive tract by eliminating some difficult-to-metabolize carbs, and in the next phase of the diet, add in small amounts, little by little, without becoming symptomatic.

TIP

The serving sizes of foods matter on the low-FODMAP diet. The low-FODMAP diet is *not* the no-FODMAP diet, so you're consuming FODMAPs in small amounts with the goal of staying under the overall amount that will cause symptoms. The Monash University app (available in mobile app stores) is a tool, created by the inventors of the low-FODMAP diet, that is used worldwide as a guide to low-FODMAP foods and appropriate serving sizes. The servings specified in the Monash University app (in green) are calculated to be under the threshold for causing symptoms, so when planning meals and snacks, make sure you don't exceed the recommended portion size.

The *stacking effect* is when multiple servings of low-FODMAP foods are consumed in a short timeframe, which increases the total FODMAPs that your digestive tract has to deal with, triggering symptoms. Keep in mind that if a food doesn't trigger symptoms one day but triggers symptoms on a different day, the stacking effect could be at play.

TABLE 8-1　**Common Foods High and Low in FODMAPs**

Category	Low in FODMAPs (Okay in Moderate Amounts)	High in FODMAPs (Avoid)
Beverages	Black tea, coffee, green tea, peppermint tea, sparkling water (plain), vodka, whiskey, wine (white or red)	Beer, chai, chamomile tea, cow's milk, energy drinks, fennel tea, kombucha, oolong tea, rum, soda (regular, diet, and prebiotic), sweet dessert wines
Cereals and grains	Buckwheat groats, buckwheat noodles, corn tortillas, cornflakes, gluten-free pasta, millet, oatmeal, polenta, quinoa, rice, rice noodles, rice puffs, teff	Amaranth, barley, couscous, kamut, rye, spelt, wheat
Dairy and dairy alternatives	Almond milk, butter (regular), coconut-based milk and yogurt, hard cheeses (cheddar, Swiss, Parmesan), lactose-free milk and yogurt, rice milk, some soft cheeses (mozzarella, feta, goat cheese)	Buttermilk, cow's milk and yogurt, ice cream, kefir, oat milk, ricotta cheese
Fruits	Banana (a few slices if ripe), blueberries, cantaloupe melon, coconut, kiwifruit, lemon, lime, orange, mandarin, passion fruit, papaya, pineapple, plantain, raspberries, strawberries	Apple, apricot, avocado (more than four slices), blackberries, cherries, dates, dried fruit, figs, grapes, mango, nectarine, peach, pear, plum, prune, watermelon
Herbs and spices	Basil, bay leaf, black pepper, cardamom, cilantro, cinnamon, clove, lemongrass, mint, nutmeg, paprika, parsley, rosemary, sage, thyme, turmeric	Dried garlic, dried onion
Legumes	Canned chickpeas (up to ¼ cup), canned lentils (up to ⅓ cup), edamame, firm tofu	Black beans, falafel, kidney beans, lima beans, navy beans, silken tofu, soybeans, split peas
Meats and other proteins	Beef, chicken, eggs, fish, lamb, pork, shellfish, turkey	Breaded or battered meat or fish, processed meats (salami, sausages), seitan
Nuts and seeds	Peanut butter, a handful of the following: almonds, Brazil nuts, chestnuts, hazelnuts, peanuts, pecans, pine nuts, walnuts	Cashews, pistachios
Sweeteners	Aspartame, maple syrup, stevia, table sugar	Agave, high-fructose corn syrup, honey, isomalt, maltitol, mannitol, sorbitol, xylitol
Vegetables	Arugula, bamboo shoots, bean sprouts, bell pepper (green, or 4 to 5 slices of red, orange, or yellow), bok choy, broccoli florets, cabbage, carrots, cucumber, eggplant, green beans, kale, lettuce, parsnip, potatoes, pumpkin, radish, seaweed, spinach, squash, tomatoes, turnip, water chestnuts, yam, zucchini (5 to 6 slices)	Artichoke, asparagus, avocado (more than two slices), beets, cauliflower, garlic, mushrooms, onion, peas, snap peas, taro

Many resources exist for helping you implement a low-FODMAP diet. The IBS-friendly recipes in this book are all compatible with the restriction phase of the low-FODMAP diet. Chapter 17 is specifically dedicated to setting you up for success if you implement this diet.

Reintroduction

The next phase of the low-FODMAP diet, over a period of six to ten weeks, is the reintroduction phase. In this phase, food categories that contain FODMAPs are reintroduced in a step-by-step manner to figure out whether you can tolerate them. This phase is important because it starts the process of making your diet less restrictive.

Generally, in the reintroduction phase, you remain on a low-FODMAP diet while purposely consuming specific foods that contain a single kind of FODMAP in increasing doses over the course of three days. If you experience symptoms, you know you've reached a level of the food your gut doesn't tolerate.

General rules for the reintroduction phase of the low-FODMAP diet are as follows:

>> Keep your baseline low-FODMAP diet as consistent as possible.

>> Each new food you consume should contain one type of FODMAP (see Table 8-2).

>> Stick to the same food for three days, with gradually increasing portion sizes of the food (tiny, small, and normal portions) over the three days.

>> Consume the food as part of a meal, rather than by itself.

>> Make note of any symptoms during the three days and in the following three days.

>> If you don't experience an increase in symptoms on any of the three days you consume the food or the following three days, you may be said to tolerate the food.

>> If you tolerate one type of food, make a note and go back to eliminating it while you test the next food.

>> Complete ten challenges (outlined in Table 8-2) to cover the FODMAP types.

>> Only after testing foods containing one FODMAP type each should you start the process of reintroducing foods containing more than one FODMAP type.

>> At the end of the process, you may reintroduce all foods that you tolerated.

If you find that a reintroduced food causes symptoms, don't be afraid to test it again later because your sensitivities may change over time. The goal is to increase the variety in your diet in a way that you can sustain over the long term.

Table 8-2 shows the ten main FODMAP types to reintroduce as you work through this phase. Choose one food from each category to test, before moving on to the next category.

TABLE 8-2 **Categories of FODMAPs to Reintroduce**

Category	Examples (Choose One to Reintroduce)	Starting Portion Size
Fructose	Honey	1 teaspoon
	Mango, diced	¼ cup
	Snap peas	½ cup
Sorbitol (polyols)	Avocado	One-quarter avocado
	Blackberries	3 berries
	Peach	One-quarter peach
Mannitol (polyols)	Cauliflower	⅓ cup
	Celery	One-quarter stalk
	Mushrooms	¼ cup
Lactose (disaccharides)	Milk	½ cup
	Plain yogurt	½ cup
Fructans (FOS), grains	Couscous	⅓ cup cooked
	Wheat bread	½ slice
	Wheat pasta	½ cup cooked
Fructans (FOS), vegetables	Garlic	One-quarter clove
	Leek	One-quarter of a medium
	Onion	1 tablespoon chopped
Fructans (FOS), fruit	Dried cranberries	2 tablespoons
	Grapefruit	One-half of a medium
	Raisins	1 tablespoon
Galactans (GOS)	Almonds	15 nuts
	Black beans	2 tablespoons
	Chickpeas	2 tablespoons

Personalization

The final phase of the low-FODMAP diet is personalizing your diet to your unique situation. This phase is key because it increases the variety in your diet and helps you meet your nutritional needs more easily and enjoyably.

As you may have found out in the reintroduction phase, even some high-FODMAP foods may not bother your digestion, allowing you to add them to your diet and eat a more diverse group of foods. In this phase, you can add all the foods you were able to tolerate into your routine. You can also experiment with other individual foods, one by one, to see whether you can tolerate them.

More than 80 percent of people who make it to this phase find they can expand their diet beyond a strict low-FODMAP regimen, providing them greater freedom in their dietary choices while keeping symptoms at bay.

MONASH: THE ULTIMATE AUTHORITY ON THE LOW-FODMAP DIET

The two scientists who published the initial groundbreaking 2008 paper outlining the low-FODMAP diet for IBS, Peter R. Gibson and Susan J. Shepherd, were based at Monash University in Australia. For this reason, Monash University is considered the birthplace of the low-FODMAP diet. Because the center has continued to investigate the diet and carry out clinical studies, it remains the world's leading authority on all things low-FODMAP.

A lab in the Department of Gastroenterology at Monash University has a range of equipment and a team of skilled staff that carry out the labor-intensive work of testing individual foods for their FODMAP content. First, the team collects the food samples for testing, including multiple samples of each food. (For each fruit or vegetable, they gather samples from ten different stores.) Then they prepare the samples by freeze-drying the edible parts and milling them into a fine powder to ensure a uniform consistency. Then the lab extracts short-chain carbohydrates from the powdered foods. Finally, they can measure the FODMAPs using a technique called *liquid chromatography*. After the FODMAP results are calculated, a dietitian determines the serving sizes that are considered low, moderate, and high.

The scientists report that a thorough analysis of the FODMAP content of just one food takes around two to four weeks in their lab. Fortunately, the information is conveniently available to people who download the Monash University FODMAP diet app, which is updated continually as the lab produces more results.

REMEMBER

The personalization phase is intended to be a long-term, sustainable diet. However, you may still need to pay attention to portion sizes and avoid the stacking effect, where you eat multiple servings of low-FODMAP foods in one sitting and thereby exceed the threshold of FODMAPs that your gut can tolerate. Over time, you'll get to know the portions that work for you.

FODMAP gentle diet

A one-phase, less-restrictive version of low-FODMAP, called *FODMAP gentle*, is considered much easier to follow while being nearly as effective for reducing symptoms. It may be ideal for people with milder symptoms at baseline. The FODMAP gentle diet emerged from Monash University, the same center where the low-FODMAP diet originated. It was advanced because of feedback that the full low-FODMAP diet was too strict for some people and may result in negative health and psychological outcomes, or it was not appropriate because of age or various health conditions.

The idea behind the FODMAP gentle diet is to restrict only common foods that have especially high concentrations of FODMAPs. The list of restricted foods are as follows, by category:

>> **Grains:** Wheat and rye

>> **Vegetables:** Onion, leeks, cauliflower, and mushrooms

>> **Fruits:** Apple, pear, stone fruits (such as peaches, cherries, plums, and nectarines), watermelon, and all dried fruits

>> **Dairy:** Cow's milk and yogurt

>> **High-protein foods:** All legumes

Some dietitians who have guided people in implementing the FODMAP gentle diet have found that excluding garlic is advisable as well, because it can lead to further symptom improvement.

After successfully restricting these foods, an individual with IBS may omit other individual foods if they're suspected to cause symptoms. So, whereas the classic low-FODMAP diet starts with more restriction and adds progressively more variety, FODMAP gentle takes the opposite approach, restricting the bare minimum and excluding more foods as required.

This diet is theorized to work in the same way as the low-FODMAP diet, but it preserves more sources of fiber in the diet, which provide nourishment for gut microorganisms that thrive on them. Symptom improvement should occur within four to six weeks at the most. The diet is typically safe to maintain over a longer term.

Gluten-free diet

The gluten-free diet for generally healthy individuals has become popularized in the past several decades. Some people with IBS try going gluten-free on their own, however, and find that it's enough to significantly reduce their symptoms. In the limited number of studies done so far, it appears that a gluten-free diet may improve symptoms that include abdominal pain, constipation or diarrhea, and fatigue.

A gluten-free diet means eliminating grains that contain the protein gluten — regular wheat, but also varieties of wheat such as kamut and spelt, as well as rye and barley. Eliminating these foods can, indeed, be effective for reducing symptoms in IBS, but surprisingly not because gluten has been eliminated. Wheat and some other grains are high in FOS, which are types of (prebiotic) fibers that the human body can't digest and that end up being broken down by bacteria in the colon. The bacterial fermentation can cause IBS symptoms. So, by eliminating gluten-containing grains, you're also eliminating a major source of gut-irritating FOS (one type of FODMAP) in your diet.

REMEMBER

Unlike with celiac disease (in which no amount of gluten is safe because it causes a damaging immune system reaction), small amounts of gluten are allowed for a person with IBS who's attempting a gluten-free diet. The effects that wheat and other FOS-containing grains have on IBS symptoms are usually dependent on the dose, so small amounts may not bother most people. But then again, if you have a gluten intolerance that affects your IBS symptoms, it may be wise to avoid all gluten. See Chapter 2 for an explanation of the difference between food allergy and food intolerance, as distinct from IBS.

If you decide to try a gluten-free diet, make sure you've ruled out celiac disease first because if you're tested for celiac disease while on a gluten-free diet, the results will be invalid. Plus, by figuring out whether you have celiac disease, you'll know for sure how strict you need to be with the gluten-free regimen.

People with IBS on the gluten-free diet should pay special attention to their intake of fiber, especially whole grains, and try to get adequate fiber intake from low-FODMAP sources. Men should aim for 38 grams of fiber per day, and women should aim for 25 grams per day. A dietitian can be invaluable for helping you figure out how to achieve this daily intake. Table 8-3 shows some gluten-free sources of fiber that are still low in FODMAPs.

TABLE 8-3   **Gluten-Free, Low-FODMAP Sources of Fiber**

Food	Approximate Serving Size	Fiber (grams)
Banana	1 medium	3.1
Blueberries, fresh or frozen	½ cup	1.8
Cabbage	1 cup	1.6
Cantaloupe melon	½ cup	0.7
Carrots	9 to 10 thick slices	0.8
Chia seeds	1 tablespoon	5
Flaxseed, ground	1 tablespoon	1.9
Green beans	10 beans	2
Oatmeal, certified gluten-free	¼ cup dry	2.2
Orange	1 medium	3.1
Peanut butter, natural	2 tablespoons	3.8

ARE IBS-FRIENDLY DIETS THE OPPOSITE OF GUT-FRIENDLY DIETS?

The purpose of adopting a diet for IBS is to reduce or eliminate gastrointestinal (GI) symptoms. However, if you compare an IBS-friendly diet such as low-FODMAP with a gut-friendly diet that's recommended for people without IBS, they seem to be on opposite ends of the fiber spectrum. Whereas IBS diets typically restrict many high-fiber foods, gut health diets actively encourage more fiber intake from a variety of food sources, especially high-FODMAP foods. This apparent paradox is because of the different aims of the two diets.

IBS-friendly diets first and foremost aim to reduce symptoms, and gut-friendly diets aim to boost the diversity and resilience of your gut microbial community and support long-term gut and overall health. The gut environments in someone with IBS and in a generally healthy person are fundamentally different, so they may react differently to fiber.

If you have IBS, you can work step-by-step: After you've implemented a diet to get your symptoms under control, you can work toward consuming more diverse sources of fiber in the diet, more akin to a typical gut-friendly diet.

Mediterranean diet

The Mediterranean diet is an eating pattern built around consuming a variety of whole foods and limiting highly processed foods with many additives. The diet emphasizes plant-based foods (vegetables, fruits, whole grains, legumes, and nuts and seeds), along with regular consumption of fish and seafood. Olive oil is used generously as the main source of fats. The diet also includes moderate amounts of poultry, eggs, and dairy products, with red meat and sweets being limited. Moderate consumption of red wine is also typical on a Mediterranean diet and may be okay for many people with IBS if they already consume wine. However, alcohol consumption in general is linked with health consequences such as liver damage, high blood pressure, and some cancers, so it's best to limit your alcohol consumption to two standard drinks per week.

Numerous studies have associated the Mediterranean diet with a longer life overall, as well as a lower risk of heart disease and other major chronic diseases. (The Mediterranean diet is definitely not the only healthy diet pattern around the world, but it's the most famous and most extensively studied by Western scientists.)

Some scientists are researching the Mediterranean diet as a feasible first-line diet for IBS (and in particular, IBS-C) when symptoms are mild or moderate. Initial research shows that people with IBS may respond to the Mediterranean diet in six weeks or less.

One randomized controlled trial from Deakin University in Australia found that when people with IBS jumped right in with a Mediterranean diet, both their GI and psychological symptoms improved, with no major shifts in their gut microbiomes. The diet may work by providing whole foods and eliminating common gut irritants found in many ultra-processed foods. Thus, the diet may have potential as a relatively easy-to-implement first option for improving IBS, especially in people who start off with milder symptoms or who initially have a diet high in sugary, fatty, and ultra-processed foods. One advantage of using this diet for IBS is that it doesn't have phases — you start off with the ultimate diet that supports health, with the aim of maintaining it over the long term.

With that said, the high intake of fiber on the Mediterranean diet may not be tolerable for everyone with IBS. A U.S. study from 2024 found that a higher intake of certain foods (fruits, vegetables, sugar, and butter) consumed as part of a Mediterranean diet were associated with more severe symptoms. Studies along these lines suggest that a standard Mediterranean diet may not be suitable for everyone with IBS and that the diet should be personalized for people who experience worse symptoms.

Other Diets for IBS Management

If you've already tried the diets in the section "Choosing a Diet to Calm Your Symptoms," or if none of them meets your needs, you may want to try one of two other diets as a possible treatment for your IBS: the low-carbohydrate diet or the high-prebiotic diet. Typically, these two diets aren't recommended as a first-line approach because they don't have a high level of scientific support, but they have been shown to work in at least some people and may be worth trying if you've exhausted other dietary options.

Low-carbohydrate diet

The low-carbohydrate diet was originally advanced as a way to lose weight by restricting the types and amounts of carbohydrates you consume. Recently, however, it has gained attention as a possible therapeutic diet in IBS-D. One study showed that within four weeks, people with IBS-D who consumed a diet containing only 20 grams of carbohydrates per day showed improvements in abdominal pain, stool form, and quality of life.

A low-carb diet restricts simple carbohydrates, such as the ones found in pasta, white bread, and sugary foods. Typical meals include meat, fish, eggs, high-fat dairy products, or leafy green vegetables, while fruits, starchy vegetables (such as potatoes and corn), and legumes are limited.

PREBIOTICS 101

Prebiotics are food for certain microorganisms in the gut that bring you health benefits. Many prebiotics are types of fiber (such as inulin, FOS, and GOS), but they can be other substances as well. Although the concept of prebiotics was first put forward in 1995, prebiotics have received more attention lately because they're one of the primary known ways to support a thriving, resilient gut microbial community.

Prebiotics in IBS are somewhat of a paradox. The most effective diet for IBS, the low-FODMAP diet, specifically excludes the most common types of prebiotics (the oligosaccharides FOS and GOS, and the foods containing them) because they tend to trigger symptoms. Yet some cutting-edge dietary approaches suggest actually ramping up prebiotic intake in IBS, with the theory that the digestive tract soon adapts, resulting in symptom improvement as well as support for the gut microbiome (see the "High-prebiotic diet" section). Plus, not everyone with IBS is actually sensitive to prebiotics in the first place, so experimenting with increased prebiotics in the diet (in foods or supplements) may be worthwhile, especially for those who experience constipation.

The low-carb diet may work in IBS by restricting many sources of FODMAPs in the diet, reducing the occurrence of symptoms. This diet may help calm symptoms and possibly also spur weight loss, but it can be hard to sustain in the long term.

High-prebiotic diet

In 2018, an interesting scientific study from Spanish scientists raised eyebrows in the IBS field. In the study, researchers compared IBS patients who adopted two seemingly opposite diets: a low-FODMAP diet versus a high-prebiotic diet. During the study, symptoms seemed to get worse temporarily for the high-prebiotic group, but then got much better as their bodies adapted. After four weeks on these diets, both groups showed reduced symptoms, except that the high-prebiotic group still experienced intestinal gas and *borborygmi* (stomach rumbling). However, when the groups stopped following the therapeutic diets, the symptoms came back immediately for the low-FODMAP group while the high-prebiotic group had sustained relief of their symptoms for two additional weeks. This sustained improvement may have been attributable to how the gut microbiota was restructured by the prebiotics, for example through increased bifidobacteria, and may indicate a healthier gut overall.

A high-prebiotic diet may be achieved using a prebiotic supplement such as inulin or FOS, or by increasing foods such as onions, garlic, and leeks in the diet. The diet may improve health overall by increasing beneficial groups of bacteria such as bifidobacteria and creating a more resilient gut microbial community. However, not everyone with IBS is willing to tolerate the possible increase in symptoms that accompanies the start of this diet. If you decide to try this diet, try to push through an initial increase in symptoms — they may reduce over time.

Avoiding Diets That Don't Serve You

In online forums for people with IBS, you'll often find someone who claims they adopted an extremely restrictive diet and saw a dramatic improvement in their symptoms. The truth about many of the extreme (and potentially expensive) regimens is that they may have worked for a specific person at a specific time, but there's little evidence that they work for the majority of people with IBS. Also, certain restrictive diets come with health risks even if they do help you keep your symptoms under control. Some of these diets can be classified as *fad diets*, which are popularized by a book or celebrity endorsement and become widely adopted by the general public despite having little to no scientific backing.

The diets in this section are not currently recommended as ways to treat IBS. Not only is there little evidence showing that they're effective for people with IBS, but they may not provide you with good nutrition if maintained for an extended period of time. *Remember:* The best chance of symptom control in IBS occurs when you start with a foundation of good nutrition and hydration, instead of eliminating most types of food.

If you decide to try one of these restrictive diets, make sure you discuss it with a registered dietitian who can guide you and help you create a plan for expanding your diet afterward.

BRAT diet

The BRAT (bananas, rice, applesauce, and toast) diet is a bland eating pattern of four foods, low in protein, fat, and fiber. This diet may be helpful for people who experience diarrhea as part of a short-term gastrointestinal infection and is sometimes used to attempt to calm symptoms (especially diarrhea) in IBS.

The BRAT diet may help some people with IBS because of the soluble fiber's bulking effect on stool, or because higher-FODMAP foods may still be tolerated by people with IBS under the right circumstances and with specific combinations of foods. The diet may not help others with IBS because both applesauce and wheat toast are high in FODMAPs and, thus, are likely irritants of the gut in IBS. The diet is excessively restrictive and, when used for more than a few days, may put you at risk for nutrient deficiencies. Different mechanisms may be at play for different individuals on the same diet, which is why no hard rules exist when it comes to diet interventions for IBS.

Carnivore diet

The carnivore diet involves restricting the entire diet to meat, poultry, eggs, seafood, fish, and water. Some people allow occasional dairy products, too. An even more extreme version of the diet involves eating only red meats such as beef and lamb. The carnivore diet is a form of the ketogenic diet, which is medically supported for people with epilepsy and type 2 diabetes. Some individuals with IBS claim this diet helped them eliminate their symptoms, which is plausible because the diet contains no FODMAPs or other fibers that typically irritate the gut in IBS.

This diet is typically not recommended because it's missing vital nutrients, and the same benefits may be achieved with more nutritional variety on a standard low-FODMAP diet. Some people with IBS use the carnivore diet with success, until they begin to feel unwell and find their health is not supported in the long term, or until they experience a side effect of the diet such as high cholesterol.

Specific carbohydrate diet

The specific carbohydrate diet (SCD) was popularized in the late 1980s with a book that described the diet as an effective treatment for inflammatory bowel disease (IBD). Since then, the diet has been studied for other gastrointestinal disorders such as IBS, but it seems to be less effective. The SCD is a grain-free diet that's low in sugar and lactose. Foods that are allowed include meats and seafood, eggs, certain legumes and nuts, vegetables (but not starchy vegetables), fruits, and honey.

The SCD, when implemented properly, is nutritionally complete. However, it may be difficult to maintain over a longer period of time.

Chapter **9**

Treating IBS with Medications

Over the past two decades, a number of medications have emerged for the treatment of irritable bowel syndrome (IBS).

TECHNICAL STUFF

IBS-specific drugs didn't begin to emerge until the early 2000s because, within the pharmaceutical industry, IBS medications were initially seen as difficult to develop. Given that no physical abnormality exists in IBS, the ideal biological target for such drugs is uncertain. As noted in Chapter 3, the underlying causes of IBS symptoms may be different for different people. Nevertheless, several types of medications have been tested and shown to be effective for subgroups of people with IBS. Some of these drugs were developed specifically for IBS, and others were developed for other disorders and found to work in certain people with IBS.

Before you consider medications for treating your IBS, two basic principles are important to understand:

» Different people with IBS have different root causes of their symptoms, so a given drug may not work for everyone. And even when a medication does work, it may have a modest effect. No IBS medication solves everything.

>> Medications are not usually recommended as a first-line treatment for IBS. Changing your lifestyle, including your diet (see Part 3), may be more effective overall with fewer side effects — an idea that's reflected in the treatment guidelines from medical associations, which recommend addressing lifestyle first and considering medications later.

Nevertheless, after lifestyle changes have been implemented, many people with IBS end up using prescription or nonprescription medications as part of their therapeutic approach. Several options for medications are available for IBS management, and a personalized strategy that considers your IBS subtype and co-occurring conditions usually leads to the best outcomes.

This chapter gives an overview of how medications fit in with overall IBS management and how to approach the use of medications. It also covers the common types of medications and supplements backed by evidence for improving IBS.

Considering Medication to Treat Your IBS

Overall, IBS treatment focuses not just on the symptoms that occur, but on the overall context of the condition: your lifestyle (including what you eat) and your frame of mind and stress levels. Indeed, evidence shows that interventions such as dietary changes (see Chapters 7 and 8) and mind-body interventions (see Chapter 11) are highly effective ways to treat IBS.

After these interventions have been implemented, you may determine (in discussion with your doctor) that adding a medication may give you additional benefits. However, figuring out which medication is right for you can be a trial-and-error process that requires some patience. Selecting medications is an art and requires taking into account your personal collection of symptoms, other conditions you may have, other medications you take, and more. You may need to try different medications in an organized sequence until you find the medication (or combination of medications) that works best for you. See the nearby sidebars for how this process may look in practice.

Deciding which medication to try

Medications can be used either to manage IBS symptoms or to modify the course of the disorder. But deciding which medication to try for relief of IBS symptoms is far from simple. No single medication works for everyone, and the best choice of medication depends on many individual factors.

MONICA'S CASE: FINDING A MEDICATION FOR RELIEF OF DIARRHEA

Monica is 28 years old and has experienced diarrhea and abdominal pain "forever," but she was finally diagnosed with IBS-D a year ago. She teaches elementary school and has limited opportunities to run to the bathroom during the day, so she limits her diet to avoid triggering diarrhea. Her diet most days consists of crackers, applesauce, and ginger ale, and she sometimes sucks on peppermint candies. Just after her diagnosis she consulted a dietitian and was found not to be a good candidate for the low-FODMAP diet (see Chapter 8), because she already avoided so many foods, which could put her at risk for nutrient deficiencies. Monica has no signs of depression or anxiety and occasionally practices yoga, which improves her symptoms somewhat. She recently took an over-the-counter probiotic for IBS for several months but discontinued it because she didn't notice any difference in her symptoms. She made an appointment with her doctor, and together they decided to proceed with drug treatment options.

First, Monica tried a 14-day course of rifaximin, which is a medication with a low risk for side effects that's intended to be taken for a short period of time. Monica didn't notice her symptoms improve during the 14 days of use, which is often expected in people with similar symptoms. However, after completing the rifaximin course, Monica noticed at the three-week mark, her stool frequency and consistency improved, as did her abdominal cramping. The doctor let her know that the symptom improvements can last a variable amount of time, from weeks to months. If the symptoms worsened again, she would be offered the choice of additional rifaximin treatments, or the opportunity to switch to eluxadoline (for which she was also a good candidate).

JOCELYN'S CASE: MANAGING CONSTIPATION

At 54 years old, Jocelyn has a diagnosis of IBS-C and experiences one effortful bowel movement every five days. She entertains friends frequently at home and enjoys wine and good cooking with a variety of fresh foods. Her kitchen cupboard is stocked with dozens of fiber-rich foods and fiber supplements, from prunes and banana flakes to Metamucil, which she has tried at various times with no improvement in her bowel movements — they actually worsen her abdominal cramps and bloating. She works in marketing and reports having an enjoyable job with moderate amounts of stress when deadlines come up. Jocelyn visited her doctor, who recommended decreasing her fiber supplement intake because of the worsening symptoms and suggested polyethylene

(continued)

(continued)

glycol (PEG) 3350 laxative, to be taken daily at first until she achieved bowel movements with more frequency along with improvements in her abdominal symptoms. The plan was then to gradually decrease the doses of PEG over time. Jocelyn tried this approach for two months and arranged a follow-up visit with her doctor to discuss the results. Unfortunately, the PEG was not effective, despite using it daily. Jocelyn still had bowel movements only every five days, and her pain was no better. The doctor recommended that Jocelyn stop PEG and start taking linaclotide. Almost immediately, Jocelyn had liquid bowel movements, something she wasn't able to recall ever experiencing, and relief of her abdominal pain. Because she noticed she had traded constipation for diarrhea, she was advised to decrease the dose of linaclotide. When Jocelyn and her doctor found the correct dose, her symptoms were much more manageable.

Many people with IBS find that they need to try out more than one medication over time to find one that works best for them. The typical approach is to start with one medication, recommended by your doctor, that seems like a good fit. Take this medication for an appropriate amount of time, and keep notes on its effectiveness. Then visit your doctor to discuss how effective it is and bring up any side effects you're experiencing. If it's ineffective, you can discuss moving on to another medication — typically, trying another drug that's in a different class, with different mechanisms of action.

TIP

Addressing every single IBS symptom through medications may not be feasible, so it's a good idea to consider what symptom bothers you the most. That way, your doctor can help you structure your management approach around that symptom. If you successfully address that main symptom, then you can look at managing the lesser symptoms next. For example, in IBS-D, after you find a medication that helps reduce your diarrhea, you may be able to use other medications as needed to reduce bloating or cramping. In other good news, some individuals find that when they address one primary symptom in IBS, several other symptoms improve without needing specific treatment.

Figuring out how often to take a medication

Some medications that manage IBS symptoms can be taken as needed, with flex-ibility around the dose and timing. For these medications, you can expect to notice for yourself how well they're working based on changes in your day-to-day symptoms. The classic example is PEG 3350 laxative for constipation: You may be able to take it daily, once every two days, or once every three days, and see what minimum level increases the frequency or softness of your bowel movements each week. You may be able to take some other medications only as needed, when your symptoms are flaring up.

Certain other medications, such as neuromodulators (described in this chapter) need to be taken exactly as prescribed because they're designed to modulate pain receptors and remodel the gut-brain axis on a lasting basis. These medications may take several weeks to months to work to their maximum potential, so they should be taken as prescribed regardless of the daily fluctuations in symptoms. Not only that, but they also may result in withdrawal symptoms if you abruptly stop taking them.

Determining whether a medication is working

When you start a new medication, take it exactly as directed. If possible, keep notes on your daily symptoms, as well as any side effects you experience, even if they seem minor or unrelated to your IBS. (You can use your phone or a written journal to track your symptoms and side effects.)

Different medications are expected to take different amounts of time to see results — some medications work immediately and others take up to two months to show benefits. After the appropriate amount of time has gone by, visit your doctor again to discuss the effectiveness and side effects of the medication. Even if a medication doesn't seem to be having the desired effect, keep taking it as directed (unless you're having uncomfortable side effects) until you're able to discuss a possible change with your doctor.

Considering cost

When you're thinking about which medication may be a good fit for you, its impact on your pocketbook may be relevant. The cost of some medications can be prohibitive. If this is the case, talk to your doctor about different options that may be available.

Addressing IBS with Medications

The number of drugs approved for use in people with IBS has expanded greatly over the years. Today, people with IBS have several options, each with its own effectiveness, mechanisms of action, and safety profile. Some of the most effective and safe medications have been incorporated into medical organizations' guidelines for the treatment of IBS.

This section covers the major categories of medications and mentions some of the common examples in each category. The generic name of the medication is written in bold.

Note that medications are generally prescribed based on the overall diagnosis of IBS, with the choice of medication depending on whether the presentation is constipation-predominant (IBS-C) or diarrhea-predominant (IBS-D).

REMEMBER

This chapter is for general information only and does not contain a comprehensive list of medications, nor does it list all side effects and precautions. Always talk with your doctor before using any medication for IBS, and follow your doctor's advice on dosage and timing. In addition, always read the product literature for any medication you take so you fully understand what the available studies have revealed about its benefits and risks. Finally, each country has its own regulations for medications available on the market, and some of the listed medications may not be available where you live.

Nonprescription medications

Some medications that are effective for IBS don't require a prescription and are available to purchase over the counter at drugstores. However, you should check with your doctor before taking a nonprescription medication regularly.

Antidiarrheals

Several over-the-counter antidiarrheals can be very useful for people who have IBS-D:

>> The drug **loperamide** acts on the enteric neurons to slow down intestinal transit, resulting in improved diarrhea. Note that gas, bloating, and pain are typically unaffected by this medication; medical guidelines don't recommend this product because of its low effectiveness. Also, some people report that after taking this product, they have difficulty achieving a bowel movement for a few days after.

>> **Bismuth subsalicylate** (or just bismuth) is a recognizable pink liquid that may improve diarrhea by increasing the amount of fluid absorbed by your intestines while lowering inflammation. This product is safe when taken in small doses for a short period of time, but toxicity may arise if it's taken over a longer term.

Both loperamide and bismuth treat symptoms of diarrhea but do not address the underlying causes of IBS. These drugs are not part of IBS medical guidelines and have limited data on their effectiveness, so they can be thought of as Band-Aid treatments to prevent embarrassing situations or resolve the symptom quickly. They don't improve the abdominal pain, bloating, or cramping that often accompanies diarrhea. Take them sparingly, and at your next appointment let your doctor know how often you're using them.

Bulking agents

Stool bulking agents, which help both constipation (by reducing stool hardness) and diarrhea (by adding volume to the stool), come in many different forms. Fiber is the best and most universal bulking agent, and you can get it through many different foods or supplements. Unfortunately, there is no one-size-fits-all approach, because everyone is slightly different when it comes to how they tolerate fiber.

Common high-fiber foods recommended for their stool bulking and/or laxative effects include

>> Bran

>> Chia seeds

>> Ground flax

>> Kiwi fruit

>> Oats

>> Prunes

Turn to Chapter 7 for tips on increasing fiber in your diet.

If foods aren't adequate for relief of constipation or diarrhea, the next step is to try higher doses of fiber through supplements. Fiber supplements are derived from natural or synthetic sources and come in a variety of forms, such as powders, pills, and gummies. Some fiber supplement products may contain sugar, artificial sweeteners, and additives, so try to choose a product with the least number of these added ingredients. Some common fiber supplements include

>> Acacia gum

>> Calcium polycarbophil

>> Inulin

>> Methylcellulose

>> Psyllium

>> Wheat dextrin

Always make sure you're well hydrated when you increase your fiber intake. High-fiber foods and supplements can sometimes worsen bloating and cramping, so if you don't tolerate higher doses of fiber, you should reduce the dose and gradually increase it over time so your body can adapt. Otherwise, try a different type of fiber. For example, inulin is a fiber that may initially lead to symptoms in some people with IBS, but if your symptoms don't improve over a few weeks, psyllium may be a good alternative. Some nonprescription products from the drugstore may also be appropriate for stool bulking or laxative effects. Not all of them are recommended in people with IBS, so talk with your doctor to find out which one is suitable. The main over-the-counter medication shown to improve constipation in IBS-C is PEG, which is an *osmotic* laxative (drawing water into the colon) for the treatment of occasional or chronic constipation. PEG is fine to use indefinitely as long as you stay adequately hydrated.

Peppermint oil

Evidence from studies around the world show that enteric-coated peppermint oil is effective for relieving both IBS pain and overall symptoms. It may work particularly well for IBS-C because menthol, its active ingredient, helps the muscles of the bowel wall to relax.

You may need to time your doses of peppermint oil carefully to see the proper effects. Normally this treatment should be taken around one to two hours before a meal, and you can work your way up from one to more doses per day as directed on the product label. Also, let your doctor know if you're taking peppermint oil for more than two weeks continuously.

Probiotics

Probiotics are live microorganisms (generally, bacteria and/or yeasts) that give you health benefits when they're taken in the correct amounts. Some probiotic products have been studied and found to bring benefits for people with IBS.

If you look at the array of probiotics available on the shelves at a drugstore or supermarket, you'll notice an array of different types, many of which have no evidence backing up their effectiveness. But a selection of higher-quality probiotic products has been studied scientifically for various symptoms or conditions, including IBS. They may bring about benefits in IBS by changing the gut microbiome and its metabolism and/or by reinforcing the gut barrier.

The effectiveness of probiotics for IBS depends on the specific strain or combination of strains. Some (but definitely not all) strains of bacteria from the groups bifidobacteria or lactobacilli may be effective on their own or in combination for improving IBS symptoms. Different probiotics may work for IBS-D, IBS-C, and IBS-M (mixed).

Probiotic products with evidence that they work for IBS include, but are not limited to, the following:

>> **VSL#3:** This combination of eight strains of microorganisms has been shown to improve diarrhea in IBS-D and reduce flatulence.

>> **Activia:** This product, with a special strain of *Bifidobacterium*, may help relieve constipation in some people with IBS-C.

>> **Align:** This strain of *Bifidobacterium* is shown to help improve gas, bloating, and abdominal discomfort, especially in individuals with IBS-D.

TIP

If you live in the United States or Canada, you can find the names of specific products for IBS in the annually updated Clinical Guide to Probiotic Products Available in USA (https://usprobioticguide.com) or the Clinical Guide to Probiotic Products Available in Canada (www.probioticchart.ca).

Prescription medications

Some IBS medications can be used only if prescribed by a healthcare professional. Several categories of prescription medications are used for IBS.

Antibiotics

An antibiotic called rifaximin, which stays within the gut and is minimally absorbed in the bloodstream, can be useful for treating IBS-D in some people. When prescribed for a 7- to 14-day course, the drug can be effective for improving IBS symptoms of diarrhea, cramping, and bloating, as well as distension. Rifaximin has few side effects and is recommended in medical guidelines for IBS. Sometimes more than one course of rifaximin is required to manage your symptoms optimally.

Rifaximin may work by shifting the gut microbial community to a more favorable composition, and by decreasing the proliferation of bacteria in the small intestine, thereby reducing symptoms in cases where small intestinal bacterial overgrowth (SIBO) is contributing to symptoms.

Antidiarrheals

Antidiarrheals may not be recommended in IBS medical guidelines because they address one symptom rather than IBS overall. However, they are sometimes prescribed because patients often find them helpful within overall IBS management.

Eluxadoline is an antidiarrheal therapy that targets the enteric nervous system, slowing down gut transit to reduce abdominal pain and diarrhea in people with IBS-D. It works on three opioid receptors in the gut, resulting in slowed intestinal motility and better pain control. This drug is recommended in medical guidelines for IBS but is not suitable for people without a gallbladder or those who drink more than three alcoholic beverages per day. Note that it's also a controlled substance and has the potential to create dependence.

Alosetron (not available in all countries) works via different mechanisms to achieve the same antidiarrheal effects. It's sometimes used for treating severe IBS-D in women, but it's generally avoided because of serious side effects, including possible *ischemic colitis* (reduced blood flow to the colon, causing tissue damage).

Antispasmodics

Antispasmodic medications work by decreasing muscle spasms in the intestines, which can be helpful when abdominal pain and cramping are the predominant IBS symptoms. Hyoscyamine and dicyclomine are antispasmodics that work by blocking the neurotransmitter acetylcholine; they may be effective for reducing pain and cramps in IBS-D. They may be limited in effectiveness, though, and are not included in IBS medical guidelines.

These medications may be available over-the-counter in some countries so be sure to inform your doctor if you're taking them for more than two weeks continuously.

Neuromodulators

Even in the absence of depression, neuromodulators (or central neuromodulators), previously called antidepressants, may be effective in IBS. Given that IBS results from altered gut-brain connections, neuromodulators can act on receptors along this axis and serve to regulate its activity by:

>> Changing gut motility

>> Improving how the brain regulates signals to the gastrointestinal tract

>> Increasing new neuron formation in the brain

>> Reducing psychiatric symptoms that may be occurring

Typically administered at lower doses than for major depression, these medications may successfully reduce pain and increase your sense of overall wellbeing. They are used for IBS-D and sometimes IBS-M (mixed).

Several different types of neuromodulators may work:

>> **Tricyclic neuromodulators,** such as amitriptyline and nortriptyline, are the most effective for relieving symptoms overall in IBS. Normally they're prescribed to treat IBS-D because they can cause constipation. Drowsiness and dry mouth are additional side effects that are frequently reported. These medications can have the positive side effect of helping with insomnia when it's a concern.

>> **Serotonin type 3 receptor antagonists,** such as mirtazapine, are particularly effective in IBS-D and in the presence of depression or anxiety.

>> **Selective serotonin reuptake inhibitors (SSRIs),** including citalopram, paroxetine, and fluoxetine are effective in some cases of IBS-C. These are not typically used as first-line therapies, but they are an option if other treatment approaches haven't worked.

Promotility agents

Promotility agents, also called *prokinetics*, are sometimes used for IBS-C because they speed up intestinal transit through increased muscle contractions in the gastrointestinal tract, thereby reducing constipation. The main promotility drug prescribed today is prucalopride, which may be used for IBS-C when laxatives are ineffective. Side effects include dizziness or tiredness.

Secretagogues

The category of drugs called secretagogues are effective for IBS-C because they increase the secretion of fluids in the intestines, making the stool softer and easier to pass. Common secretagogues include the following:

>> **Linaclotide** is an effective secretagogue for treating IBS-C. Anyone who takes the drug may run the risk of severe diarrhea, so the dose may need to be adjusted.

>> **Tenapanor** improves IBS-C by acting on the surface of the small intestine and colon to block absorption of sodium in the intestine, resulting in increased sodium and phosphorus retention within the intestine and, thus, softer and looser stools. This drug is especially effective for decreasing bloating and may reduce abdominal pain.

>> **Lubiprostone** increases chloride secretion into the intestinal lumen, speeding up intestinal transit and increasing fluid content, resulting in softer stools in people with IBS-C.

JUST SAY NO TO NARCOTICS FOR IBS

When symptoms won't go away, some individuals with IBS may receive a prescription for narcotics (opioids) such as codeine, morphine, meperidine (Demerol), or hydromorphone (Dilaudid) to reduce pain and diarrhea. These substances may relieve pain and improve diarrhea by slowing gut motility, but longer-term studies show that they ultimately lead to worse outcomes. Not only do they carry a risk of serious side effects (such as difficulty breathing and severe drowsiness), but they're also highly addictive. As if that weren't enough, they can result in a condition called *narcotic bowel,* which worsens constipation and pain perception. One UK study found that one-fifth of people with IBS received a prescription for opioids, and that being prescribed such drugs was associated with more severe symptoms, a lower quality of life, and increased costs for managing their IBS. Overall, narcotics are best avoided in IBS treatment. Their ideal use is for short-term pain management, such as after surgery, not for a chronic condition.

Chapter **10**

Exploring Emerging Treatments for IBS

When medical doctors recommend treatments for irritable bowel syndrome (IBS), they have standards for what they recommend: typically, they want to see evidence from more than one scientific study showing that the treatment is safe and that it works for people with IBS. The treatment approaches described in Chapters 7 through 9 and in Chapter 11 meet these standards.

If you talk with other people who have IBS or follow them on social media, you may discover that some of them have great confidence in treatments that *don't* meet these high standards of evidence. One person may say that the occasional shot of Jägermeister made all the difference to their symptoms, while another person may say that regular ice baths helped them gain control over their IBS. Others may put their trust in a multi-herbal supplement they bought online. Even though these unconventional strategies may not work for most people with IBS, each of them clearly worked for at least one person, so they can't be dismissed outright.

There's merit to keeping an open mind about the kinds of IBS treatments that may work. Although scientists know a great deal about effective IBS treatments from research over the past three to four decades, many of them recognize the limitations of existing treatments and the gaps in understanding the underlying causes of IBS, so they continue their research with the aim of finding better therapies. Currently, IBS is understood as a cluster of symptoms that show up for diverse underlying reasons, including visceral hypersensitivity, altered gut microbes, abnormal motility, and more (see Chapter 3). So, it's highly possible that some treatments work well across the broad population of people with IBS, and other treatments work only for a subset of people with IBS who have a specific combination of biological and lifestyle or environmental factors. Over time, unraveling all these factors will help advance personalized medicine.

In the meantime, people with IBS have the option of choosing some treatments that are less rigorously researched. This chapter covers some commonly used emerging treatments for IBS — that is, treatments that don't (yet) have a lot of evidence backing their use. Some of these treatments are frequently supported by anecdotes or testimonials found in marketing materials or on social media, or even through word of mouth. The aim of this chapter is not to dissuade you from trying these treatments (as long as they're safe and appropriate for your type of IBS), but rather to encourage you to be aware of the potential limitations.

REMEMBER

If you decide to try one of them, you should still discuss it with your healthcare provider. With an organized and deliberate approach, you'll be open to the treatment's possible benefits while being cautious of the potential downsides. At the end of the day, regardless of whether an emerging treatment turns out to be effective, the goal is to end up smarter about your IBS and how your body works.

Understanding Evidence for Treatments

Evidence-based treatments for IBS are those that are supported or informed by a sufficient amount of objective evidence from scientific studies. More specifically, these treatments have been tested in groups of people with IBS, ideally in a controlled study where one group receives the target treatment and another group receives another treatment, and neither group knows which group they're in until the study is over. Personal stories are not evidence because they don't take an organized and unbiased approach to answering whether the treatment works for the population of individuals with IBS.

REMEMBER

When little to no scientific evidence shows the effectiveness of a treatment, it can't be considered evidence-based. When a small amount of evidence supports a treatment's benefits, it may be called *emerging*. All evidence-based treatments started off one day as emerging treatments and gained their evidence-based status over time as more studies were completed. So, yes, tools may be added to the toolbox of evidence-based treatments as the years go by. But at this moment, people with IBS can benefit from what scientists know based on the best available proof, giving them the best chance of success and helping them to avoid wasting time and money on approaches that don't work.

Thus, at this point in time, a basic contrast exists between evidence-based and emerging treatments for IBS. When you come across a new potential treatment online or in a health-food store, here are some ways to know if the treatment is emerging:

>> It's not usually recommended by doctors or other mainstream medical professionals.

>> It's not covered or reimbursed by national or personal health insurance.

>> A search of scientific articles — for example, in PubMed (https://pubmed.ncbi.nlm.nih.gov) — brings up few or no studies on it.

>> Only one company sells the product, and there's no obvious way to contact that company to find out what evidence supports the product's effectiveness.

TIP

Before trying one of these emerging treatments, here are some questions to ask yourself:

>> How do I know this treatment is safe and won't make my symptoms worse?

>> How much benefit do I reasonably think this treatment will bring me?

>> How much time and money does the treatment cost? Can I afford it?

>> Who is recommending this treatment? What is their professional background to make such recommendations? Do they benefit financially if I try it out?

>> What knowledge will I take away even if the treatment doesn't work for me?

If your answers give you no cause for concern, then going ahead with the emerging treatment may be worthwhile.

REMEMBER

You should discuss with your doctor each treatment you want to try *before you try it*. This way, you can make sure the treatment is appropriate for your diagnosis, doesn't interact with existing medications, and won't make other medical issues worse.

Digging into Emerging Treatments for IBS

You don't have to look very far to find emerging (or non-evidence-based) treatments for IBS. From the supplements website that trumpets the "one and only solution" for bloating or pain, to the social media influencer who gives you precise instructions for a miracle smoothie, many sources offer up treatments that haven't been rigorously tested and may or may not turn out to be effective. This section walks you through some of the emerging treatments you may come across and what to know before you try them.

Taking dietary supplements

Dietary supplements are products consumed to enhance the diet — usually either a natural or synthetic version of a substance found in foods.

The key thing about dietary supplements is that, as dietary add-ons, they're primarily aimed at healthy people. (Regulations that apply to dietary supplements are slightly different around the world, but in general, manufacturers of dietary supplements can't claim that a product treats or improves a diagnosed disease, because to do that, a product must be a medication.) Thus, supplement labels may not specifically mention IBS, even if they're intended for use in people with IBS.

In the following sections, we cover the various types of dietary supplements you may want to consider for IBS.

Herbal supplements

Herbal supplements are dietary supplements containing one or more herbs or plants. Herbs can be consumed in teas or taken in pills that provide a larger and more controlled dose. The following herbal supplements are commonly used for IBS symptoms:

>> **Aloe vera:** Aloe vera is a cactus-like plant with a thick liquid inside the leaves that can be used on the skin or ingested in supplement form. It's thought to be anti-inflammatory, with possible laxative effects in those with constipation. In the few studies that exist, aloe vera appears safe and shows a possible benefit for IBS symptoms.

>> **Anise:** Anise is a flowering plant with a licorice-like flavor, used in traditional Persian medicine. At least one study showed that coated anise oil capsules were effective for reducing IBS symptoms in people with IBS. Licorice root, which has a similar flavor, is also sometimes used as a digestive aid. Note that overuse of these herbs may put you at risk for increased blood pressure problems or electrolyte imbalances.

>> **Curcumin:** Curcumin is a spice with anti-inflammatory effects, and some studies show that it may help abdominal pain and improve quality of life in IBS. It has also been shown to modulate the gut microbiota.

>> **Fennel:** Fennel is a vegetable that has been used for thousands of years for both culinary and medicinal purposes. Its seeds are commonly used as an after-meal digestive aid in India and other countries. Fennel has possible anti-gas-formation properties and may reduce abdominal pain in people with IBS. Several studies found that a combination of essential oils from both curcumin and fennel, taken in pill form, improved symptoms and quality of life in people with IBS.

>> **Ginger root:** Ginger root is the rhizome of a flowering plant, often used fresh or as a dried spice in cooking. Extracts from ginger root, when taken in capsule form, may be helpful for reducing inflammation. A growing group of studies show that ginger or ginger root extract helps reduce IBS symptoms, with particular reductions in bloating, gas, and diarrhea.

>> **STW-5:** This is a multi-herbal preparation that has several potential effects, including on gastrointestinal (GI) motility, intestinal permeability, and the gut microbiota. STW-5 is safe for the liver and may be effective for improving IBS symptoms.

Biotic supplements

Biotic supplements are supplements with the *–biotic* suffix: probiotics, prebiotics, synbiotics, and postbiotics. Specific supplements within all these categories are said to help with IBS, with varying levels of evidence. Here's what to know about each type of biotic:

>> **Probiotics:** Probiotics are live microorganisms that offer health benefits when they're consumed in the correct amounts. Many products are labeled as probiotics when they're not the real thing. Probiotics backed by evidence must have at least one study showing they give a health benefit; the exact health benefit depends on the probiotic strain or combination of strains, so products are not interchangeable. Some probiotics have convincing evidence that they can reduce symptoms in IBS, so they're included in Chapter 9. But the majority of probiotics available on the market are *not* shown to work in IBS (although you may try them and see some benefits).

>> **Prebiotics:** Prebiotics are substances that certain gut microbes consume to give you a health benefit — in other words, they're food for beneficial microbes. Many prebiotics are varieties of dietary fiber, but other substances can be prebiotics as well. Chapter 9 covers prebiotics proven to work in IBS. Other prebiotic products are available, which may or may not be effective

for IBS. However, prebiotics may be worth trying out, especially in IBS-C (constipation). Note that prebiotic side effects may include nausea, bloating, and worse abdominal pain, but these tend to improve over time.

>> **Synbiotics:** Synbiotics are made up of two parts — live microorganisms and food for live microorganisms — which work together to bring you a health benefit. Some synbiotic combinations are shown to be effective in IBS and are promising for further study.

>> **Postbiotics:** Postbiotics are substances that contain dead or inanimate microorganisms (with or without the metabolites they produce), which bring about health benefits. Relatively few studies have been done on postbiotics, and confusion exists within academia and industry around the word *postbiotic* because an older definition referred to only the metabolites of gut microbes. Postbiotics have been used for many years in Japan, and several specific postbiotics are being studied for immune benefits. However, some postbiotic products have been shown to reduce GI symptoms in IBS.

REMEMBER

The general rule when it comes to biotics is that each one should be individually tested for effectiveness in IBS. For example, even though one probiotic strain may be effective for reducing symptoms, a closely related strain may not be effective at all. Sometimes combinations of strains are found to be more effective for IBS than single strains.

Other supplements

Some non-herbal supplements also constitute emerging treatments for IBS:

>> **L-glutamine (glutamine):** Glutamine is an amino acid, used to create proteins, and it's found in food and also produced in the body. It's believed to have a role in gut barrier integrity and changing the gut microbial community in a positive manner. Limited evidence so far shows glutamine may have benefits for symptoms in IBS; one study showed that supplementing with glutamine enhanced the effectiveness of a low-FODMAP diet.

TECHNICAL
STUFF

FODMAP stands for fermentable oligosaccharides, disaccharides, monosaccharides and polyols. Read more about a low-FODMAP diet in Chapter 8.

>> **Magnesium:** This nutrient helps regulate blood pressure, heartbeat, and bone strength. It may relax the muscles of the digestive tract, and it's sometimes used to relieve constipation in IBS.

>> **Melatonin:** Melatonin is a natural compound produced by your body and also by outside sources, and it's recognized for its role in controlling sleep-wake cycles. Across several studies, melatonin has been found to improve IBS symptoms, including abdominal pain. It may also have beneficial effects on sleep parameters in people with IBS.

Understanding fecal microbiota transplantation

Fecal microbiota transplantation (FMT) is a treatment that involves transferring *feces* (stool) from a healthy person into the colon of another person. It's no joke — this unconventional-sounding treatment has been investigated for dozens of different conditions that are understood to be linked to the gut microbiota. The theory is that FMT replaces a disrupted gut microbiota with a healthy microbial community from the donor.

Of all the conditions that FMT has been investigated for, it seems to work reliably only for recurrent *C. difficile* infection — that is, a GI bacterial infection with *Clostridioides difficile* that *recurs* (comes back) despite multiple courses of antibiotics. This success led to standardized FMT products approved by the U.S. Food and Drug Administration (FDA) being available in the United States.

To date, the studies on FMT have shown mixed results for improving IBS, but this treatment is being actively studied to see if the success rate may be improved.

Only certain individuals may respond well to this treatment. FMT may change the gut microbial community of the recipients with IBS, even if it doesn't improve their symptoms.

WARNING

Importantly, as with any other treatment, risks exist with FMT, especially when the donor stool is not thoroughly screened for infectious and antibiotic-resistant microorganisms. (For this reason, FMT should not be attempted at home.)

Despite the cautions against FMT, several studies around the world continue to investigate it in clinical trials as a treatment for severe IBS. In the future, researchers may discover a subgroup of people with IBS who respond well to FMT, or they may develop a more targeted and safer version of FMT that's consistently effective in IBS.

Trying other treatments

Other treatments that fall under the category of emerging are antihistamines, digestive enzymes, neurostimulation, and acupuncture.

Antihistamines

Common over-the-counter medications called *antihistamines* block the effects of histamine, which is produced in the body or consumed in food. Normally used to reduce allergy symptoms, antihistamines may also help relieve abdominal pain and bloating in IBS — particularly in the IBS subgroup whose symptoms are driven by histamines (see Chapter 2).

Digestive enzymes

Digestive enzyme supplements such as FODZYME are specifically designed to break down the major FODMAP sources in the diet (fructan, galacto-oligosaccharides, and lactose) for better digestion and lower gas production. Evidence suggests that these supplements may reduce certain symptoms, although consumer reviews are mixed.

Neurostimulation

Neurostimulation is a treatment that involves electrical stimulation directly targeting nerves in the brain. Various areas of the brain can be stimulated via electrodes on the surface of the skin. The aim is to affect the areas of the brain that process pain, thereby reducing abdominal pain in IBS. Little research has confirmed whether this treatment is effective in IBS.

Acupuncture

Acupuncture is a treatment that originates from traditional Chinese medicine in which a skilled technician inserts thin needles into the skin at precise locations. The needles stay inserted for a period of time while the individual rests, and then they're taken out. Initial studies show that acupuncture may provide benefits to some people with IBS — so if you find that it works for you, regular acupuncture treatment may be something to try.

Navigating Emerging Treatments

When you decide to start an emerging treatment, it's best done in a deliberate manner to ensure that no matter what happens, you gain some knowledge and move forward in your IBS journey. Here are some important actions to make sure you derive the maximum benefits from the treatment:

>> **Don't start multiple treatments at the same time.** Make sure you leave about a month between the start date of different treatments, to get a sense of which one is actively working for you.

>> **Where possible, don't invest a lot of money up front in an emerging treatment.** For example, avoid signing up for monthly mail order probiotics; instead, try a trusted brand from a health-food store.

>> **Adhere to the directions for the treatment you choose and stick to a consistent schedule.** Follow the instructions on the label. In addition, write down how much and how often you take it, and the date you started.

>> **Keep a symptom record.** Jot down your symptoms a few days before starting the treatment, and continue through the first days and weeks after you start the treatment. Consider sharing this record with a healthcare professional to help you identify any patterns.

>> **Monitor other health problems.** If you notice that any health issue gets worse after you start the treatment, even if it seems unrelated, stop taking it and see whether the issue resolves. Report this information to your health-care provider.

REMEMBER

By keeping good records, you can learn something from every treatment you try out for IBS symptoms.

What if you find an emerging IBS treatment that works well for you, and you're passionate about telling others how it helped you? That's great! In addition to telling your story, try to find ways to help move evidence forward on the treatment — for example, by helping raise money to fund research studies.

SUPPLEMENTING WITH A DOSE OF HOPE

Hope can be powerful — especially in a disorder of gut-brain interaction (DGBI; see Chapter 2) such as IBS. A boost of positive emotion in people with IBS is sometimes associated with fewer symptoms. Hoping that a treatment will work can lead to the *placebo effect,* which is a benefit that occurs not because of the treatment itself, but because of a belief that a treatment will work. But why not put the placebo effect to work for you? Studies show that it can have real biological effects that could potentially benefit IBS symptoms. So, maintain a positive outlook and keep the hope alive when you try out a new treatment, and you may actively improve your health in the process!

Chapter **11**

Seeking Mind-Body Treatments

I f you have irritable bowel syndrome (IBS), you're living proof of the close connection between the gut and the brain — and more specifically, the power of your brain to influence your physical symptoms. The most up-to-date understandings of IBS acknowledge that the condition is a disorder of gut-brain interaction (DGBI), in which the two-way communication between the digestive tract and the brain is disrupted. So, it's no surprise that psychological stress or excitement can be a major trigger of symptoms, even when no obvious gut stimulus (such as a trigger food) is present.

But here's the good news: You can use the gut-brain connection to your advantage. By working to calm your brain through mind-body treatments, you can succeed in reducing your gut symptoms and increasing your quality of life.

Mind-body treatments (or mind-body interventions) are a set of brain retraining techniques promoting *neuroplasticity* (reorganization of brain connections). They go beyond simple calming or relaxation and actually retrain your brain, through various mechanisms and signals, to regulate both brain and body functions. The main practices are cognitive behavioral therapy (CBT), yoga, breathing, meditation, and gut-directed hypnotherapy.

These interventions are the missing piece in many people's IBS treatment regimens, and a lack of brain-focused treatments is a frequent reason for being unable to get IBS symptoms completely under control. Because the main symptoms of IBS show up in the gut, many people understandably focus on gut-centric treatments such as diet. However, they may be overlooking brain-related treatments, even though the latest research on IBS clearly shows that the best outcomes occur when an individual targets both the gut and the brain simultaneously. Mind-body interventions are backed by more research than most people realize — in fact, the research is so convincing that many countries' national guidelines for IBS management now recommend considering psychological treatments targeting the body, or mind-body treatments.

This chapter covers the rationale for mind-body treatments, as well as the mechanisms of how they work, and explains the specific interventions that are shown to work well in IBS. By implementing one or more of these techniques, you'll be able to put mind over matter in getting control of your IBS symptoms with a set of skills to use for physical and mental wellness.

Understanding Why Mind-Body Treatments Work

The importance of targeting the brain has long been understood in IBS care — for example, medications such as neuromodulators have been used for IBS management because they target the central nervous system and autonomic nervous system pathways to achieve pain control. But medications ultimately have limited effects on the psychological factors that contribute to IBS, making mind-body interventions a necessary addition to a comprehensive treatment approach.

On the whole, mind-body interventions in IBS are thought to restore the balance between the *sympathetic* (fight-or-flight) and *parasympathetic* (rest-and-digest) nervous system responses, thereby optimizing the function of the enteric nervous system, including gut motility and secretions. Mind-body interventions also appear to reduce perceptions of pain by improving the invisible connections between brain structures, as well as by modifying the physical structures of the brain to decrease perceptions of fear, anger, anxiety, and hypervigilance. Moreover, mind-body interventions are for the most part safe and feasible, and unlike medications, they invite individuals to actively participate in maintaining their own health and develop a sense of ownership over their own well-being.

Most mind-body interventions are ideally practiced on a daily basis for people with IBS. At the outset, they require guidance by a qualified instructor (preferably one with experience helping people with digestive disorders) to ensure safety and to personalize the approach, and later they can be practiced at home. The recommended minimum practice varies by activity. The research on yoga, for example, supports an optimal duration of 20 minutes per day, at least three times a week, with more practice resulting in a greater treatment effect. For other mind-body interventions, a qualified professional may advise on the frequency of practice.

Most people with IBS are very open to trying mind-body interventions, with about 30 percent naturally adopting these practices through their own reading and investigation. Even more individuals adopt these techniques following a recommendation from their physician. They don't require a certain level of performance or experience. However, some people may feel restless if they're new to these practices or may find the exercises boring. If this sounds familiar, working in person with an experienced practitioner or guide may help you focus your mind more effectively, making the practice more enjoyable.

Mind-body interventions work quickly, with most people seeing results within about 30 days of starting. The response is usually moderate but long-lasting, so if you implement a mind-body intervention, you may retain the benefits even 6 to 12 months afterward.

Choosing an Effective Mind-Body Treatment

Several mind-body interventions backed by scientific studies are described in this section: CBT, mindfulness techniques (breathing practice, meditation, mindfulness-based stress reduction [MBSR], and yoga), and gut-directed hypnotherapy. By implementing one or more of these treatment approaches, you may be able to reduce the unpredictability of your symptoms or decrease their occurrence overall.

Dozens of studies, with thousands of total participants, have investigated various mind-body treatments for people with IBS and shown them to be effective for reducing symptoms. Few studies have done a head-to-head comparison of one mind-body intervention versus another, however, so it may be best to pick one of the approaches that's suitable to integrate into your lifestyle, and observe the personal difference it makes. Intentionally modifying your lifestyle to accommodate an intervention requires commitment and habit development, but it frequently results in a durable response over time.

Committing to cognitive behavioral therapy

CBT is based on the simple truth that your thoughts and feelings affect how you behave. Negative thoughts may lead to negative emotions, causing you to behave in undesired ways. Particularly for people who have IBS, these negative patterns can become entrenched in brain activation circuits, with undesirable gut and brain symptoms occurring in a seemingly never-ending cycle.

CBT is a type of psychological therapy in which you retrain your brain and unlearn the negative thoughts and behaviors that have developed around your gut symptoms and stress. By developing a more positive outlook and broader perspective on your IBS and the rest of your life, you can powerfully affect how you behave and manage IBS. CBT has been demonstrated to work by optimizing the brain connections, otherwise known as the *connectomes*, that activate and deactivate various regions — ultimately leading to better pain management.

Typically, someone with IBS learns CBT for a short term. Over a series of sessions with a qualified CBT practitioner, you learn techniques such as *cognitive restructuring* (identifying unhelpful thought patterns and changing them) and *behavioral change* (adjusting your thinking and behavior to different circumstances).

These skills help you manage stress as well as negative thoughts and emotions (fear and anxiety, for example). Specifically, a well-designed CBT treatment may decrease the severity and frequency of your IBS symptoms; it may also improve your quality of life while addressing symptoms of anxiety and depression.

CBT is the mind-body treatment that has been the most frequently studied and currently has the most evidence for effectiveness in IBS (although other mind-body interventions may develop more evidence over time as they continue to be studied). CBT has a better success rate than most available IBS medications, without side effects, and it may work well for people who haven't responded to medications. It can even be delivered effectively in group sessions or via phone or online. Some centers are also experimenting with delivering CBT through virtual reality. However, only a small number of people with IBS receive CBT in practice. Possible barriers include the availability of a qualified practitioner and the cost of treatment.

Cultivating mindfulness

Skills to develop mindfulness help you calm your mind and body simultaneously, helping you cope with stress as well as gut-based symptoms. When you develop mindfulness, you're directing your attention to what's happening in the present moment while letting go of all thoughts about the past and worries about the future. Mindfulness involves being aware of what you see, hear, smell, touch, or taste in the here and now — that is, intentionally making yourself focus on the current moment. Mindfulness also includes accepting all your thoughts and emotions without judgment and letting them pass. The underlying theory of using mindfulness in IBS is that by keeping yourself grounded in the present moment, even if you have pain or discomfort, you'll be more accepting and you'll let go of all the baggage around that discomfort. You may also be more likely to deal with the discomfort in a constructive way. Mindfulness is an excellent tool for combating stress, because it helps you focus on changing the stressful environment or implementing a strategy to reduce stress. Mindfulness is shown to lead to significant improvements in the severity of IBS symptoms, a better quality of life, and less pronounced anxiety.

Several helpful practices encourage you to cultivate mindfulness: breathing, meditation, MBSR, and yoga. Each of these has the benefit of restructuring your brain to help you be more at ease, both overall and when you experience IBS symptoms.

Breathing

Breathing is an activity you need to do to stay alive — but it's so much more than that. By using certain breathing techniques, you can activate the rest-and-digest functions of your body (via the parasympathetic nervous system) and fix the disruption in homeostasis that's brought about by stress. Certain breathing techniques are designed to stimulate the *vagus nerve*, which helps your body shift toward parasympathetic responses. The vagus nerve conveys sensations to the central nervous system and alters areas of the brain such as the thalamus, limbic areas, and anterior cortical areas, ultimately reducing your experience of pain.

More than a hundred breathing techniques exist, any of which can lead to benefits when practiced for just a few minutes per day. If you have IBS and you're new to breathing techniques, alternate nostril breathing, diaphragmatic breathing, and box breathing are good exercises to focus on. The latter two are described in this chapter. During some yoga classes, you may also learn breathing techniques that may be applied in your life off the mat.

TIP

Start by learning some of these breathing techniques from a professional (ideally a yoga therapist with expertise in digestive health) to maximize their effectiveness and safety. In your daily life, when you become excited or stressed and you feel your breath becoming fast and shallow, these breathing techniques may be accessed in that moment, helping your body come back into a relaxed, nonstressed state.

People with IBS may find that a good approach is to set aside time in their day (perhaps 10 minutes) to practice breathing techniques. For best results, you need a calm setting, preferably an empty gastrointestinal tract, and you need to sit or stand with good posture. One favored breathing exercise for many people with IBS is called *diaphragmatic breathing*, also called *belly breathing*. This technique involves consciously slowing and deepening your breaths for an instantly accessible state of calm.

Your *diaphragm* (a muscle situated under your lungs, running along the bottom of your rib cage) is employed in diaphragmatic breathing to give a gentle massage to your internal organs. Here are the basics of how to practice diaphragmatic breathing:

1. **Take a seated position with good posture.**

2. **If you're new to diaphragmatic breathing, place one hand on your chest and the other hand on your belly, just under your ribs.**

3. **Slowly breathe in, and try to keep the hand on your chest steady as the hand on your belly gently rises with the breath.**

4. **Slowly breathe out, and notice the hand on t belly gently falling as your belly draws inward.**

   Engage your diaphragm muscle to push out the air in a strong and steady manner.

5. **Repeat the cycle of breathing in and out for around ten breaths, inhaling for the count of four and exhaling for the count of six.**

   In other words, your exhale should be just slightly longer than your inhale.

Some people with IBS-D (diarrhea) say that diaphragmatic breathing can help with the panic that comes when they feel pain and urgency with no bathroom in sight. And others with IBS-C (constipation) say that practicing diaphragmatic breathing while on the toilet can help them relax and engage the proper muscles for an easier bowel movement.

Box breathing (also known as *square breathing*) is another technique, which is practiced as follows:

1. **Take in a slow, deep breath through your nose for a count of four seconds.**

2. **Hold your breath at the top of the inhale for four seconds.**

3. **Slowly exhale through your mouth for four seconds.**

4. **Hold your breath at the bottom of the exhale for four seconds.**

5. **Repeat the pattern for several cycles.**

Meditation

Meditation is a practice that involves training your attention and awareness and detaching from automatic, unfocused thinking. The cliché of sitting cross-legged and clearing your mind is only one of the possible ways to practice meditation. Various meditation practices include:

>> Breath awareness meditation

>> Mantra meditation

>> Silent meditation

>> Sound meditation

>> Spiritual meditation

>> Transcendental meditation

Many tools exist to help you develop a meditation practice. Most people with busy, active lives find it difficult to jump right into effective meditation — and that's okay. Meditation is a practice you develop over time. Start small, guided by a professional or perhaps with a validated app or video that can take you through a short meditation sequence. Over time, breathing exercises and attentional focus will strengthen your body, mind, and energy systems to prepare you for more impactful meditative experiences. Meditate in the morning if possible before you jump into all the activities of your day, with ten minutes being a good length to aim for.

TECHNICAL STUFF

Studies have shown that mindfulness meditation increases the activity of gamma-aminobutyric acid (GABA) receptor neurons, also known as *GABAergic neurons,* in the brain. These special neurons help create breathing rhythms and help increase the communication between respiratory and cardiac areas in the medulla. They also help control activity that excites the amygdala, an area of the brain with a big impact on anxiety behaviors. In one IBS study, an eight-day intensive meditation program increased mindfulness while creating changes in the participants' resting brain connectivity, as shown through *functional magnetic resonance imaging* (fMRI), a noninvasive brain imaging technique that measures brain activity through blood flow changes. In other words, the changes in participants' mindfulness scores were correlated with signs that people had trained their brains to function differently.

Mindfulness-based stress reduction

MBSR is a specific program that helps you calm your mind and body to better manage stress and pain. In one study, more than 70 percent of people with IBS who took part in an eight-week class on MBSR experienced a noticeable reduction in their symptoms. In particular, those who increased their ability to stay focused on the present moment and act with awareness were more likely to show improvements in their IBS. Other studies showed a particular improvement in quality of life in people with IBS who undertook this intervention. You can access MBSR through a psychologist, social worker, or other health professional who has completed specific MBSR training.

Yoga

Yoga is a practice that originated in India thousands of years ago. It involves a series of physical poses, as well as meditation and controlled breathing. Its aim is to unify the body, mind, and spirit.

Yoga has become increasingly popular in the Western world, having moved into the mainstream around the 1970s. Today, it's estimated that around 21 million adults in the United States have practiced yoga within the past year.

Yoga is known to benefit both generally healthy people and those with IBS. Yoga has multiple effects, including less perceived stress, mood improvements, reduced blood pressure, and regulation of blood sugar. The beneficial effects of yoga come from multiple components put together: deep breathing, meditation, and physical postures. These three activities serve to influence the gut–brain axis by:

» Reducing the activity of the sympathetic nervous system (fight-or-flight)

» Increasing the activity of the parasympathetic nervous system (rest-and-digest)

» Modulating the function of the hypothalamus-pituitary-adrenal axis (involved in stress responses)

» Improving brain connectivity by modulating connectomes and by producing cannabinoids and dopamine (feel-good hormones)

» Increasing GABA concentration in the brain, which inhibits excited or anxious feelings

TECHNICAL
STUFF

Regular yoga practice changes the structure and function of the brain. Imaging studies have found increased gray matter in the insula and hippocampus, as well as increased activation in prefrontal areas of the cortex, with regular yoga practice. In addition, increases in function occur in the frontal executive and attention areas, which are responsible for planning and organizing your behavior.

For people with IBS, yoga may decrease both physical symptoms and mental symptoms. Its efficacy appears comparable to CBT. A study by one of this book's authors, Dr. Raman, examined an eight-week program with weekly virtual yoga classes plus home practice for people (mostly women) with IBS. The classes included physical postures, breathing exercises, mantra meditation, and breath-watching meditation. The average participant attended a weekly virtual class and practiced for 21 minutes per day. The severity of IBS symptoms significantly decreased in the yoga group but didn't decrease in a control group that received advice only. In addition, the yoga group fared better than the control group on quality of life, fatigue, and perceived stress.

Many different styles of yoga exist, which are distinguished by the postures and their sequence, the pace of the postures, and their spiritual basis. Any type of yoga can give you benefits, but remember that the benefits don't just come from the physical postures. They come from all three components together — the postures, the breathing, and the meditative focus. Research is underway to identify IBS-specific yoga postures for maximum effectiveness.

A large study on yoga safety found that it was safer than other exercise types, but there was a small risk of musculoskeletal pain or injury. However, three-quarters of people who experienced pain or injury made a full recovery, and the risk of injury decreased greatly when practicing with a qualified yoga instructor or yoga therapist.

Exploring gut-directed hypnotherapy

Hypnosis, once merely a parlor diversion in Victorian society, has made a big comeback among the general public. The number of people using hypnosis apps is growing quickly, and YouTube hypnosis videos featuring swirling patterns and candles have logged tens of millions of views.

Hypnosis has made a comeback in the medical world, too. Evidence shows that hypnosis is a useful clinical tool in many domains: chronic pain or headaches, sleep problems, smoking cessation, and mental health issues such as anxiety and phobias. Gut-directed hypnotherapy is a highly effective mind-body intervention for improving IBS. The aim of gut-directed hypnotherapy is to achieve greater focus and awareness while in a relaxed state, which helps your brain change its activation pattern and, thus, alter your experiences with IBS.

By now, a convincing amount of high-quality evidence shows that gut-directed hypnotherapy is effective for reducing or relieving IBS symptoms (abdominal pain, bloating, gas, nausea, and stool consistency) and improving quality of life for people with IBS, no matter what their IBS subtype. The success rate is around 70 percent to 80 percent, with the effects being immediately apparent. And remarkably, after a successful program of gut-directed hypnotherapy, some people report that the effects are maintained months and years later — a better track record than all the available medications for IBS. One caveat for this intervention, however, is that it's most effective for people whose mood symptoms (anxiety and depression) are controlled.

In gut-directed hypnotherapy, a qualified practitioner guides you in a safe and comfortable manner into a special mental state (hypnosis). This state enables you to go beyond your conscious thoughts to access your subconscious mind, which invisibly controls thoughts, emotions, and behaviors. The practitioner delivers standard gut-directed suggestions, as well as personalized suggestions, with your subconscious mind becoming open to the gut-healing suggestions and soothing imagery delivered during the session. You remain aware of what's happening the entire time, and when you come out of the hypnotic state, you may see lasting improvements in the communication between brain and gut, with positive effects on your symptoms. Gut-directed hypnotherapy can address the physical and emotional effects of stress, as well as negative thought patterns and somatic symptoms that are common in IBS.

TECHNICAL STUFF

Gut-directed hypnosis works by modulating the gut-brain axis in a lasting way. Studies have shown post-hypnosis biological changes that lead to positive changes in gut-brain function: normalized gut motility, reduced visceral pain perception, and restoration of normal pain processing in the brain.

Gut-directed hypnotherapy comes in many forms: in-person classes, online classes (individually or in a group), or via an app such as Nerva (https://try.nervaibs.com) or LyfeMD (www.lyfemd.ca). People who completed a program of gut-directed hypnotherapy on a popular app daily were shown to have comparable results to those who had in-person sessions.

Integrating Mind-Body Techniques into Daily Life

Feeling stress may be an inevitable part of life, but how you react is fully under your control. If people with IBS fail to pay attention to managing their stress they're likely to end up with worse gut symptoms. So, individuals with IBS need to become pros at eliciting the relaxation physiological response as discussed in this chapter in order to keep gut symptoms under control.

To best manage your IBS, stay aware of your stress and your response to it. Making a commitment to practicing some form of mind-body treatments regularly will help you normalize your biology and mental wellness and reduce your symptoms.

Fortunately your options for accessing mind-body interventions are many. Some people choose to seek out a class, while others find videos or apps helpful. Nerva is a well-known app for gut-directed hypnotherapy, while LyfeMD has a highly effective yoga/breathing/meditation program specifically for IBS.

TIP

Here are some tips for integrating mind–body techniques into your daily life:

» Start your day with a regular practice of yoga, meditation, or breathing, before other activities get in the way. End your day with a similar practice.

» Aim for just a short practice so you can keep it up day in and day out (and consider adding it to your digital calendar).

» Vary your practice (perhaps alternating between yoga and a sitting meditation, for example) to keep up your interest.

» Become an expert in at least one breathing practice that you can implement on demand during stressful or anxiety-provoking circumstances.

» Keep a recording of your favorite meditation practice at hand, so you can listen while driving, doing errands, or when you have a moment alone.

» Consider including a gratitude practice in your routine.

The final goal is to be able to access the mind–body calming techniques whenever stress arises in your daily life. With regular practice, you'll be able to pull out the strategy you need right at the moment you need it.

TERRI'S CASE: MIND-BODY INTERVENTIONS FOR THE WIN

Terri is a 41-year-old single mother of two children, ages 6 and 8. She works as a part-time administrative assistant and cleans houses on the weekends. For the past year, she's had increased stress and anxiety because of family issues after her mother's death, and she has experienced bloating and distension as well as alternating constipation and diarrhea. Terri received an IBS diagnosis recently. Given her current stressors, Terri's family physician prescribed a neuromodulating agent (amitriptyline). She was advised to adopt a low-FODMAP diet, but after learning more about it, she declined this approach because of the added mental burden and lack of capacity for behavior change at this point in her life. She was certain that her IBS was worsened by stress rather than diet, and she was eager to learn strategies for stress management. Terri was recommended a holistic multicomponent yoga program that included postures, breathing, and meditation. She attended weekly in-person classes and practiced at home on the other days. Within just 30 days, her stress and anxiety had improved dramatically, leading to improvements in her IBS symptoms.

Chapter **12**

Adjusting Your Lifestyle to Manage IBS

What's your favorite daily habit? Is it a cup of coffee you have in the morning, or perhaps a hot shower? Is it the moment you take to sit and cuddle with a pet, do a word puzzle on your phone, or put on your fuzzy slippers in the evening? Any of these habits are part of the overall picture of your lifestyle, and they may have both physical and psychological importance to you.

Lifestyle is a concept that's expansive and somewhat hard to define. In a basic sense, your lifestyle is the total collection of your habits and behaviors, as well as your overall living conditions. Some of these things you consciously choose, and others are dictated by circumstances. Lifestyle includes both the broad strokes (such as whether you live alone or with other household members) and the details (such as how often you wash your hair and which shampoo you use). All the details of your life come together to create your unique lifestyle. Even two people living under the same roof may have aspects of their lifestyles that are completely different from each other.

To be clear, your lifestyle is different from what marketers mean when they refer to a "lifestyle brand" or a "lifestyle store." In those cases, lifestyle is an aspirational state of having certain products around you. But lifestyle in general is more than just a cute set of ceramic mugs and 500-thread-count sheets. It's everything about your day-to-day living — the good, the bad, and the non-aesthetic.

Your lifestyle has thousands of parameters that fall into patterns as you exist on a day-to-day basis. The power of lifestyle factors when it comes to your health is that they're modifiable, in contrast with many health-related factors that are not modifiable, such as your genes.

REMEMBER

Your lifestyle is the most significant — and perhaps the most daunting — factor you need to address when it comes to managing your irritable bowel syndrome (IBS). It includes both diet and mind-body practices, which are so important that we discuss them on their own in separate chapters. (See Chapters 7 and 8 for information on diet, and Chapter 11 for information on mind-body treatments.)

This chapter covers other aspects of lifestyle and their potential to impact IBS symptoms. First, the chapter covers why lifestyle is so important for IBS management. Then it goes through the specific lifestyle changes that may help you manage your IBS. Finally, the chapter presents a step-by-step plan for implementing lifestyle changes and making them stick. The specifics are different for each person, but after reading this chapter, you'll have a good idea of how you're able to adjust your own lifestyle for better control over your IBS.

Understanding How Your Lifestyle Impacts IBS

With some diagnosed disorders, you can start taking a specific medication to correct a biological imbalance and then more or less carry on with the life you're living. IBS is different, though. IBS is a complex disorder of gut-brain communication with no single underlying cause, so it requires a holistic approach that includes lifestyle modification. Only by controlling certain daily habits and overall behaviors do you have the best chance of finding relief from your IBS symptoms.

Does paying attention to your lifestyle mean you need to control every single aspect of your daily life with IBS and make your habits completely predictable? No. It just means you need to be aware of your habits and fine-tune the ones that aren't working for you.

Take Paul, for example: He loves streaming action shows, and when he gets caught up in a new series, he tends to stay up late, streaming episode after episode on his computer and falling asleep in front of the screen. This results in sleep deprivation and makes his IBS symptoms worse. Paul doesn't have to stop binge-watching altogether when he finds a good show, but he can start watching the episodes earlier in the evening and shut off the computer before bed, perhaps implementing a non-screen activity such as reading or doing a short meditation before he falls asleep. Using similar approaches, you can preserve the activities you enjoy while reducing the impact on your IBS symptoms.

In the bigger picture of IBS management, your lifestyle factors are often hiding in plain sight. That is, the details of your lifestyle may seem so normal and inevitable that changing them may never have even occurred to you. But after you become aware of certain lifestyle factors, you may be surprised to find that you can successfully change them, and that your IBS symptoms respond very positively to those changes.

Becoming aware of your lifestyle

When you want to make lifestyle changes to reduce the impact of IBS, the first step is being aware of your lifestyle. Many people are so accustomed to their routines that they're unaware of all the details of their lifestyle. No two people have exactly the same lifestyle, so this is a personal reflective exercise that only you know how to do. Here are some questions to think about, which will help you get a sense of what your unique lifestyle is like:

>> Do you live alone or with other household members? What's your relationship with them? Do you have a role in caring for them?

>> If you engage in paid work, how many hours per day do you spend working? How would you describe your work-life balance?

>> What's your typical mode of transportation when going from place to place?

>> What's the total income for your household? What are your main expenses?

>> What's your general health status? When was your last doctor's appointment and dental appointment?

>> What medications or supplements do you currently take?

>> How many hours per day do you sleep, and what's your sleep like?

>> How much time each week do you spend outdoors? Do you use sun protection?

>> What do you typically eat in a day? How often do you consume alcohol?

>> Do you smoke or vape?

>> How active are you, and what physical activities do you undertake regularly?

>> Which wellness appointments do you regularly attend (for example, acupuncture or massage) and how often?

>> Do you spend time on hobbies? How often do you socialize with people outside your household?

Questions such as these can help you understand what defines your lifestyle in this current time and place, and spark ideas about what factors may be impacting your IBS symptoms — even if you currently take those factors for granted.

Knowing the limits of lifestyle change

Not everything about your lifestyle can be changed at any given time. Because of responsibilities or other factors, every person has certain limits to the lifestyle changes they can reasonably implement. For example, a busy parent at home with three young children may want to find time to meditate daily but may have difficulty finding time to use the bathroom privately, let alone meditate. Or someone working as a nurse in a hospital intensive care unit (ICU) may have certain job demands that limit their ability to control stress.

With that said, better awareness and tools can help you overcome perceived barriers, and in some cases it's possible to change the limitations that exist. Sometimes you can make big or small decisions that have an important impact on both your lifestyle and your ability to manage your IBS. The parent at home with children may be able to hire a babysitter one afternoon per week and do a meditation exercise (among other things) during that afternoon. Perhaps the nurse can apply to transfer to another part of the hospital where the job involves less urgency and stress than the ICU.

Certainly, big decisions such as a job change shouldn't be taken lightly — before you decide to do so, you may want to write out the pros and cons as well as the possible impact on others in your life. You may also seek help from a coach or therapist to gain a clearer perspective on your life and prioritize among all your complex responsibilities. Sometimes with a little creativity — or bravery — you can overcome apparent limitations to change your lifestyle in ways that help you get a handle on your IBS symptoms. You may end up feeling more empowered, leading to a better quality of life overall.

Identifying which lifestyle factors to change

After you're aware of your lifestyle and how much it can realistically be changed, the next step is to identify which lifestyle factors are having an outsize impact on your IBS symptoms. These are the factors you can focus on changing as part of your IBS treatment plan.

The lifestyle factors that typically make a difference for IBS are diet (see Chapters 7 and 8) and controlling stress and mood through mind-body treatments (see Chapter 11). Other powerful lifestyle factors are described in this chapter's sections, "Making Lifestyle Changes to Manage Your IBS" and "Building Good Lifestyle Supports for Managing IBS." Meanwhile, some other factors that help your IBS may not be found in these pages because they're personal to you.

Making Lifestyle Changes to Manage Your IBS

Apart from diet and stress/mood management, studies consistently show that certain lifestyle factors can make a big difference in the symptoms of people with IBS. These main factors are physical activity, sleep, and staying healthy by avoiding infections. Another minor lifestyle factor — adjusting your toilet position and technique — can also make a difference for some people with IBS.

Committing to exercise

Exercise is purposeful physical activity that you undertake to improve your health. Incorporating regular exercise into your routine is one of the most effective lifestyle changes you can make when you have IBS. On the other hand, some people with IBS find regular exercise difficult because it seems to trigger their symptoms.

Overall, some people with IBS say diet modification is the best way to keep their symptoms under control, but others find that exercise alone is enough to improve their symptoms (with research showing 20 minutes of daily walking may be as beneficial as yoga and the low-FODMAP diet put together). But in all cases, exercise should be considered alongside the other interventions you're implementing for IBS.

TECHNICAL STUFF

FODMAP stands for fermentable oligosaccharides, disaccharides, monosaccharides and polyols. Read more about a low-FODMAP diet in Chapter 8.

Across studies, increased exercise or physical activity is shown to have the following impacts for people with IBS:

>> Reducing gastrointestinal (GI) symptoms

>> Improving cognitive symptoms and mood

>> Improving quality of life

REMEMBER

For people with IBS, the best exercise involves regular, moderate-intensity physical activity — for example, a daily walk of 20 to 30 minutes, a relaxed ride on a stationary bicycle, or some swimming. Shooting a basketball, dancing, or gardening also hit the optimal zone of moderate physical activity. Both tai chi and some forms of yoga may be helpful because of their meditative components and controlled breathing along with the physical movements. Around 20 minutes a day is adequate in most cases, but if you can't manage that much on some days, even a few minutes of exercise is better than none.

WARNING

More strenuous feats such as long runs, spin classes at indoor cycling studios, or high-intensity interval training (HIIT) should be attempted with caution by people with IBS because heavy exertion may draw blood away from your digestive system, which can cause diarrhea and other uncomfortable symptoms. (If you're an athlete who undertakes more strenuous exercise on a regular basis, refer to Chapter 16.)

You also need to find a type of physical activity that's feasible and enjoyable for you to do on a regular basis. For example, you may love visiting the climbing gym, but if the nearest location is an hour away, visiting regularly may not be practical. Conversely, you may live next door to an excellent pool facility, but if you hate swimming, you probably won't be successful in keeping up the habit.

Choosing a type of exercise you can do outdoors or in nature may have additional benefits for mood and stress relief. However, access to toilet facilities may be a factor in the type of exercise you select. If you walk outdoors for exercise, you can use a toilet-finder app to make sure you know where the available toilets will be along your route, just in case the need arises. When you find an activity that fits well into your routine and that you look forward to doing, you'll know you've found the right activity for your lifestyle.

TIP

If exercise seems to trigger your symptoms, try to work your way up to a regular routine of physical activity. If you're new to exercise, you may try walking outdoors or on a treadmill with controlled breathing for just a few minutes and gradually increase the time to 20 minutes daily. At first, you may want to walk with a friend or family member for support. The important thing is to make the activity a regular habit. Persistence is worthwhile because the research is clear: People with IBS who practice regular, moderate-intensity exercise are better off in the long term.

Achieving good sleep

A good night's rest is one of the key lifestyle factors that can make a difference for IBS. Not only can poor sleep worsen your IBS symptoms, but it may also make you drowsy and accident-prone, interfere with thinking and memory, and worsen your mood. Poor sleep is linked with chronic health conditions such as heart disease, obesity, type 2 diabetes, dementia, and some cancers.

THE FART WALK GOES VIRAL ON SOCIAL MEDIA

Canadian actress and cook Mairlyn Smith is known for encouraging people to consume more fiber in their diets, but she acknowledges that fiber can have an unpleasant side effect: increased intestinal gas. In a video on social media, Smith shared one of her top tips for "aging wonderfully" and lessening the discomfort of intestinal gas. She explained that every day, around one hour after eating dinner, she and her husband go on a 20-minute stroll that they call a "fart walk" to help digestion and release pent-up gas in the gut. Some scientists, seeing the proliferation of the hashtag #FartWalk on social media, weighed in, and they agreed that exercise after a meal can be very helpful for releasing gas that's contained in the digestive tract. Not only that, but a post-meal stroll can also help relieve constipation and normalize blood sugar levels, leading to healthier metabolism.

If you like the idea of a fart walk but can't get out of the house after dinner for one reason or another, you may be able to use a treadmill or stationary bicycle to help your digestion move along. Or grab your yoga mat and do some gentle stretching, or put on a good tune and dance like no one's watching!

Three important factors to consider about your sleep habits (also called *sleep hygiene*) are as follows:

>> **Sleep duration:** How long you sleep

>> **Sleep continuity and quality:** How uninterrupted your sleep is (which impacts sleep quality, or the stages of sleep that impact restfulness)

>> **Sleep timing:** What times of night or day you sleep

Sleep that's shorter, interrupted, or out of sync with your body clock may worsen your IBS symptoms. Most people need to sleep between seven and nine hours every night, waking up briefly no more than twice (or not at all), to feel rested and alert throughout the day.

Here are some proven tips for good sleep hygiene:

>> **Go to bed and get up at a consistent time each day.** Consistency can help your body establish its *circadian rhythm* (that is, the body's internal 24-hour clock). For best results, try to stick to the pattern even on the weekends or other days when you're outside your usual schedule.

» **Avoid caffeine in the afternoon and evening.** Caffeine can make you feel alert for a short time when you actually need sleep, so limit your caffeine intake as much as possible every day throughout the afternoon and evening.

» **Turn off the screens at least 30 minutes before bed.** Laptops and phones emit blue light, which promotes wakefulness and makes falling asleep more difficult. The National Sleep Foundation suggests replacing screen time before bed with a restful activity such as a warm bath, reading a book or magazine, listening to music, or meditating. Quiet conversation with a household member may also work.

» **Establish a bedtime ritual.** Doing the same activities day after day before bedtime can help signal to your body that it's time to wind down for sleep. For example, every night before bed you may change into your pajamas, brush your teeth, put on some calming music, and read for a few minutes in a comfortable chair. This ritual may trigger physical and mental relaxation processes that help you fall asleep more quickly.

» **Reduce your bedroom temperature by a few degrees overnight.** If you wake up often during the night, try reducing the room's temperature. A cooler space mimics the drop in body temperature that occurs while you sleep, so your body has to put less effort into cooling you down.

» **Create a completely dark sleeping area.** Another thing that may be waking you up at night is light, so try to eliminate all sources of light in your bedroom. Use blackout blinds around windows or cover the edges of the blinds with towels while you sleep. And don't forget to turn off the alerts on your electronic devices and place them in a location where you won't see them lighting up.

» **Reduce noise while you sleep.** If you find yourself being awakened by noises during the night, try using a white noise machine to drown out other sounds. You can also consider wearing earplugs or a soft headband that covers your ears.

» **Take melatonin or magnesium before bed.** Melatonin supplements may help signal to your body that it's time to sleep. And recent studies suggest that melatonin may have benefits for IBS symptoms, too. Magnesium supplements may also help you sleep by promoting muscle relaxation.

» **Experiment with naps.** If you have difficulty staying alert throughout the day, see if you can incorporate a 20-minute nap into your schedule. A brief nap may help you manage your energy levels and function better during the day. However, some sleep experts advise against naps because they may interfere with your quality of sleep at night. You may need to experiment to see what works best for you.

Note that hormonal fluctuations may also affect sleep; these fluctuations may be important to address with your doctor, especially in females approaching menopause. If you have good sleep hygiene and you still aren't feeling rested upon waking, you may have an undiagnosed sleep disorder. Talk with your doctor about what you're experiencing and see if further testing is warranted.

Avoiding infections

Getting exposure to a wide range of microorganisms in your daily life — for example, by spending time outside in nature — is a good thing. But the microorganisms you want to avoid are the ones that specialize in causing infections that could harm your health. When certain types of bacteria, fungi, viruses, or parasites called *pathogens* gain access to your body, they may multiply and interfere with your normal biological functioning.

Avoiding infections is important for two reasons:

>> **Dealing with the infection itself can be unpleasant.** For example, GI infections often cause diarrhea, nausea, and vomiting. Or infection with the SARS-CoV-2 virus (also known as COVID) can lead to extreme tiredness, coughing, shortness of breath, body aches and pains, and other symptoms. Your IBS symptoms may overlap with these infection symptoms, and you may suffer more in the short term.

>> **GI infections can sometimes lead to (or worsen) IBS-like systems that persist for a long time after the infection goes away.** When this occurs, you may have post-infectious IBS.

TIP

The upshot is that avoiding infections in your everyday life is highly worthwhile because it can prevent numerous problems in the present and the future. These are some of the top evidence-based ways to reduce your risk of infections that may harm your health:

>> **Wash your hands frequently with soap and water.** This advice is repeated so often that it's easy to dismiss, but washing your hands every time you get the opportunity is a highly effective way to avoid the spread of infectious microorganisms. Definitely wash your hands after using the bathroom and before eating, but also when you get home from an outing, after blowing your nose, and after shaking hands with people or touching pets. (Make sure you have a good lotion nearby, too, because all the handwashing can make your skin feel dry.)

>> **When you're in a public place, avoid touching your face and consider wearing a mask.** Your eyes, nose, and mouth are key points of entry for

infectious microbes, so touching these areas puts you at risk for an infection to take hold. Furthermore, some infections are spread through the air so it may be prudent to wear a mask when traveling or in very crowded places.

» **Practice good food-sharing hygiene.** When you take a sip from someone else's drink or use a communal pile of ketchup in which someone has double-dipped, you risk sharing saliva-borne germs. Instead, use only clean dishes and cutlery and dish out food and condiments individually.

» **Practice good food safety.** The skins of some fruits and vegetables can harbor harmful bacteria, so make sure you wash them well before you consume them, especially if they aren't going to be cooked. Peeling the skin off fruits and vegetables after washing is another good practice (although it may reduce the amount of dietary fiber you consume). In addition, make sure to handle raw meats safely and cook meats to the recommended internal temperature. Keep cold foods cold to prevent the growth of harmful bacteria.

» **When you have a cut, wash it, dry it, and cover it with a bandage.** Some pathogens can infect you through cuts in the skin. A lesion on the skin is at risk of getting infected if it's not clean or if you touch or pick at it, so be sure to protect it with a bandage.

» **Stay up to date on your vaccinations.** The evidence is clear: When public health vaccination programs for a disease are implemented in an area, the incidence and complications of that disease go down sharply. The safety of vaccines is also continually monitored by governments and health organizations. Make sure you receive the vaccines recommended by your local health authority in a timely manner. And when you plan to travel, book a travel vaccine appointment several months in advance and receive any shots that are recommended for the place you're visiting.

» **Avoid contact with wild animals.** Animals that live in the wild often harbor microorganisms that are unfamiliar to humans and may cause harm — for example, bats often carry the virus that causes rabies. Thus, avoiding direct contact with these animals is advisable. Also, when infections are known to be circulating within domesticated animal populations, it's best to avoid contact with those, too. (Farmworkers may need to take extra precautions during these times.)

Toilet position and technique

Sitting on the toilet and straining to have a bowel movement is among the more frustrating activities you can do, and it's not an uncommon activity for people who have constipation as a symptom of their IBS.

DEALING WITH FATIGUE

Do you often feel you don't have the energy to do everything you need or want to do? Fatigue during the daytime is quite common for people with IBS — in fact, it's the third most common non-digestive complaint. Those who are younger and female may report fatigue more frequently. In addition to getting a good night's sleep and adjusting eating patterns to stabilize energy throughout the day, here are some tips for reducing fatigue:

- Stay hydrated.

- Consume adequate levels of nutrients overall in your diet.

- Get regular exercise.

- Practice breathing exercises during the day and before bed.

- Make sure depression and anxiety are treated appropriately.

- Treat any other medical conditions that you may have.

- Get help or assistance with your daily tasks when needed.

If you implement these techniques and you're still tired, you may need to adjust your expectations about what you can reasonably accomplish during the day. Consider what your priorities are (or should be) and try to put most of your energy into the high-priority activities. If you're not sure how to do this, talk with an occupational therapist, who can give you personalized advice on strategies for conserving energy in your daily routines and completing your most important daily activities.

Unfortunately, standard Western toilets aren't ergonomically designed to allow the easiest bowel movements. But fortunately, you can adjust your position on the toilet for better success. By elevating your feet using a special toilet stool, you assume a squatting position that allows your muscles to better help you go. One popular brand is the Squatty Potty (www.squattypotty.com).

Another thing you can do to engage the right muscles during a bowel movement is to push out your breath in a focused manner. Some people liken this technique to blowing bubbles through a straw — and if it helps, you can even blow air through a real straw that you hold in your mouth. Alternatively, you can think about blowing out a candle. Either way, this technique activates the vagus nerve and triggers the muscles of digestion as well as the wavelike muscle movements called *peristalsis* that help push substances through the digestive tract.

Building Good Lifestyle Supports for Managing IBS

In addition to daily habits, you may be able to build some other activities into your lifestyle on a regular basis to support your IBS management. This section doesn't contain a comprehensive list, but it may give you some ideas for regular services that help support your wellness with IBS over the long term.

Massage

Massage is manipulation of the body's soft tissues for therapeutic purposes. In IBS, massage can be helpful on different parts of the body. For example, a full-body relaxation massage can reduce stress overall and relax the body physically, helping to alleviate symptoms. More specialized massages may address digestion or mood specifically. Abdominal massage can be especially helpful for people with constipation, because it can relieve tension in the abdominal muscles, reduce cramping, and stimulate the normal digestive processes. A registered massage therapist is the best person to seek out for a safe and effective massage.

TIP

Self-massage is massage that you do on your own body. Abdominal self-massage can be relaxing in a general sense; it can also help stimulate better bowel movements in people with IBS. Consult with a registered massage therapist for instructions personalized to you and your symptoms.

DISTINGUISHING BETWEEN IBS AND PELVIC FLOOR DYSSYNERGIA

IBS is distinct from a condition called *pelvic floor dyssynergia*, which involves incoordination of the pelvic floor muscles. For example, if you have constipation, you may inadvertently develop the habit of bulging the abdominal muscles while contracting the pelvic floor, working against a successful bowel movement. Some people may even experience *pelvic organ prolapse*, in which the wall of a pelvic organ such as the rectum or vagina bulges into an adjacent space. Pelvic floor therapy may alleviate some of these problems and establish good muscular habits during bowel movements. In addition, people with diarrhea may have bowel urgency or incontinence if they lack strength or functional control of their pelvic floor muscles; this may also be addressed through pelvic floor therapy. Talk with your doctor if you think you may have a problem related to the pelvic floor, in addition to IBS.

Physiotherapy

Physiotherapy is not routinely recommended in IBS, but it may be helpful if you have pelvic floor dyssynergia, pelvic organ prolapse, or fecal incontinence along with IBS.

Your body's pelvic floor has muscles that help control bowel movements. A successful bowel movement requires contraction of deep abdominal muscles along with full relaxation of the pelvic floor muscles, and these muscles may function incorrectly in some conditions.

Here are some activities that a physiotherapist may include as part of pelvic floor therapy:

» Education about pelvic floor anatomy and function and bowel control mechanisms

» Pelvic floor sensation and motor control exercises

» Electromyographic (EMG) biofeedback therapy, which uses electrodes on certain muscles to generate a feedback signal (for example, on a screen) when the muscle contracts

» Pelvic floor exercises that you can integrate into daily activities (for example, coughing, sneezing, rising from sitting, or standing)

Implementing Lifestyle Changes That Stick

When you identify the lifestyle factors you'd like to change to get a better handle on your IBS, successfully changing them may be another matter altogether. Say you want to exercise more regularly. If you intend to fit in the exercise when you have free time, you may never find that free time in your day. Willpower takes you only so far. Instead, exercising must become a habit — for example, exercising every day right after breakfast in the morning, or as soon as you get home from work. When you get into a routine, you won't overthink it, and you'll find that the exercise becomes less effortful.

TIP

Overall, here's what experts say about the process of making your chosen lifestyle changes stick:

» **Set a goal for what you want to change.** Pick one main goal and articulate exactly why you want to change this aspect of your lifestyle. To set your goal, you may want to ensure it follows the principles of SMART: specific, measurable, achievable, realistic, and timely. For example, "I will exercise for 30 minutes, three times per week for the month of March, to boost my energy levels so I can socialize more with my friends." It may be helpful to write this goal on a card where you'll see it every day.

>> **Put your plan in place.** To achieve your goal, you may need various resources as well as a plan for making it happen. First, figure out how you'll get the resources you need, whether that's a comfortable pair of walking shoes or certain foods. Then make specific plans on how to make it happen.

REMEMBER

Establishing new habits may take time and patience. If your goal is to walk 30 minutes per day, start with a shorter walk and work up to the target length over a few weeks. Creating new habits works best when they're triggered by something that occurs during your day. For example, you may set a daily alarm that reminds you to exercise, or place your running shoes by the dog's food dish so right after you feed the dog you remember to put them on and go for a walk.

>> **Find an accountability buddy.** If you have a good friend who's willing to help hold you accountable, establish a way to communicate about your lifestyle goals and check in (perhaps weekly) about whether you're meeting them.

>> **Stay focused on the positive.** As you're working to establish a new behavior, you may experience setbacks. Don't give up if you skip a few days for one reason or another. Expect that you may have difficulty establishing the habit at the beginning stages, but know that if you persist, you'll be in a much better position.

REMEMBER

Positivity breeds success. Write down the benefits you see, and try to change negative thoughts such as "This is too hard" to more positive ideas such as "This is hard and I can do hard things." Some people may find it useful to gamify their goals; if you're one of them, look for an app that helps you set goals and gives you digital rewards when you meet them.

>> **Think through the barriers you may face.** Even before you begin, plan ahead for possible barriers to meeting your goal. Factors such as fatigue, pain, a busy schedule, and more can get in the way of making the changes you want. Jot down your plan for each possible barrier. For example, "If I feel too tired to go for a walk, I'll put on my running shoes and do ten squats." (After you have your running shoes on and do the squats, you may just feel like walking after all.)

>> **Evaluate success and reset goals after the previous goals have been achieved.** After a period of time, evaluate the progress you've made toward your goal. If you haven't met the goal, take a look at where you started and how far you've come. Celebrate yourself for coming that far and push onward. If you've completely met your goal, consider setting another one!

NICK'S CASE: THE VIRTUOUS CYCLE OF LIFESTYLE CHANGES

Nick, a 40-year-old male with IBS, was in a self-described slump. For the past ten years, he'd had occasional IBS symptoms that didn't particularly bother him. But two years ago, he lost his job and he still hadn't been able to find stable employment. During those two years, he gained 30 pounds and his IBS symptoms were continually flaring up, with abdominal cramping and diarrhea. The family dynamics and financial situation were altered — Nick's wife, a schoolteacher, was now the main income earner. When Nick sought out his doctor's help, he reported feeling depressed and having three or more bowel movements per day, accompanied by abdominal pain and excessive intestinal gas.

A closer look at Nick's lifestyle habits revealed that he drank around eight cups of coffee per day, along with three cans of soda and three to four bottles of beer. He spent most of his time in the house, with very little physical activity. Nick was advised to undertake a step-by-step lifestyle plan: First, he cut down his intake of caffeinated and carbonated drinks to one coffee, one soda, and one beer per day. After two weeks, he was able to eliminate these beverages altogether and drank water as his sole source of fluids. In the weeks that followed, Nick lost 15 pounds just by eliminating the extra calories in the various beverages. This encouraged him to be more active, getting outside for short daily walks. The exercise improved his outlook and prompted him to see a psychologist for help with stress management. He developed techniques for more positive thinking and was able to direct more energy toward looking for a new job. Along the way, his IBS symptoms greatly diminished. By addressing multiple aspects of lifestyle one by one, Nick eventually got his symptoms and his life under control. Nick's case shows how one positive lifestyle change can lead to another, with success leading to more success in a virtuous cycle.

Chapter **13**

Maintaining Your Quality of Life with IBS

One TV ad about a product for irritable bowel syndrome (IBS) likened digestive symptoms to an annoying friend (or frenemy, perhaps) named Irritabelle who follows you around, demanding your attention at the absolute worst times. Irritabelle, it seems, has a knack for knowing exactly when her intrusion will be the most inconvenient and never fails to ruin your plans. "Who makes the decisions around here?" she says to the person with IBS, holding up a finger in warning. "It's me."

Many people with IBS will see some truth in this depiction: Even after they implement a variety of treatment strategies (diet, lifestyle, and medications) and stick to them as much as possible, their symptoms still trail after them and sometimes cause unpredictable disruptions. This can interfere with your quality of life.

REMEMBER

Any efforts to improve your quality of life should take into account both your symptoms and your overall environment, including the places you frequent and the people you have around you. This chapter offers lots of tips — it's up to you to decide which ones are suitable for your personal combination of symptoms and your environment. By employing the appropriate strategies, you may feel more confident and give yourself the gift of a better quality of life.

TIP

The top factor for improving your quality of life with IBS is improving your social contact and supports. Even though socializing can feel daunting at times when you have IBS, it's important that you try to maintain relationships with at least a few close friends or family members. You don't have to be the world's biggest extrovert, but you should take time to regularly connect with a few people whose company you enjoy. You can be creative about when and how you communicate, but make sure you maintain the relationships for the sake of your own wellness.

This chapter offers some insider tips for improving your quality of life when you live with ongoing IBS symptoms.

Finding Tools and Services for IBS

With IBS being so prevalent across the population and with awareness of the condition increasing, a host of new tools and supports have emerged specifically for helping manage it. Entire companies have focused on specific IBS solutions, such as apps or snack foods, and many healthcare professionals specialize in helping people with IBS.

WARNING

One caveat: Not all the products and services marketed for IBS will work for you. Maintain a healthy skepticism and think about how a solution may fit into your overall lifestyle before you spend your money.

Using technology

A growing number of purpose-made smartphone apps may help you manage your IBS more effectively. Some provide comprehensive tracking of your symptoms and lifestyle habits; others focus on specific types of information and reminders. Here are some of the apps that exist for people with IBS (search the App Store or Google Play Store for the app's name, or visit the following links to learn more):

>> **IBS Coach** (`https://ibscoach.org`): This app simplifies the process of implementing a low-FODMAP diet by providing meal plans, symptom tracking, and coaching. It includes a four-week program designed to identify food triggers and improve symptoms.

TECHNICAL STUFF

FODMAP stands for *fermentable oligosaccharides, disaccharides, monosaccharides and polyols.* Read more about a low-FODMAP diet in Chapter 8.

>> **LyfeMD** (`www.lyfemd.ca`): This digital platform offers evidence-based holistic and behavioral approaches to digestive health management, including diet advice, mental wellness programs, and health coaching services.

WHAT IS QUALITY OF LIFE?

Quality of life is a measure of your perceived well-being at a certain point in your life. It isn't about an objective standard that applies to everyone. One person's idea of a good quality of life might be living in a cozy, quiet home and having friends or family over for regular Friday movie nights. But for another person, a good quality of life may mean living downtown and going to a nightclub every weekend. Quality of life relates to your personal goals and lifestyle and may include how often you have to change your behaviors and plans because of your illness. A high quality of life doesn't mean eliminating all the tough times, but it means structuring your life so you have meaning and purpose beyond those tough times.

For people with a high quality of life with IBS, the following statements are true:

- You feel at ease and empowered in your daily life

- You take part in the activities you want to

- You feel good about your body most of the time

- You feel you have reasonable control over your health

- You generally enjoy food

- You're satisfied with the healthy sexual relationship(s) you have in your life

- You feel socially accepted and have close supporters who you can talk to about your IBS

If IBS symptoms are getting in the way of any of these factors, then IBS may be reducing your quality of life. Fortunately, you can take action to help improve on this measure.

» **Monash University FODMAP Diet (**www.monashfodmap.com/ibs-central/ i-have-ibs/get-the-app**):** This gold-standard app for the low-FODMAP diet features a way to look up the FODMAP content of different foods, giving you confidence as you plan your meals. The app also has a wealth of information about IBS and the low-FODMAP diet, as well as a built-in diary for tracking your diet, symptoms, and more.

» **myIBS (**https://cdhf.ca/en/how-to-use-cdhfs-myibs-app**):** This is a health diary app for people with IBS, which allows you to digitally track symptoms, bowel movements, food, sleep, stress, and other factors, to help you better manage your IBS on a daily basis. The app also allows you to share progress with friends.

» **mySymptoms Food Diary (**www.mysymptoms.net**):** This app has a flexible daily food and symptom tracker, which can help you figure out which foods may trigger your IBS symptoms.

» **Nerva: IBS & Gut Hypnotherapy** (https://try.nervaibs.com): This unique app uses hypnotherapy to address the gut-brain axis and manage IBS symptoms. The six-week program of guided hypnotherapy sessions may have positive effects on stress and reduce its effects on IBS symptoms.

» **Spoonful** (https://spoonfulapp.com): This app helps you read labels on food products and can tell you if a product is high or low in FODMAPs.

TIP

Several apps can help you find available public bathrooms that you can use while you're out and about. Just search your smartphone's app store for "toilet finder."

Finding services

Where can you find professional services to help you manage your IBS? It depends on where you're located and the model of care, but here are a few places to look for different types of services:

» **Gastroenterology:** The American College of Gastroenterology (ACG) website (https://gi.org) can direct you to resources and help you find a gastroenterologist in your area. In addition, some large, well-known medical institutions feature IBS centers of excellence, with many professionals under one roof.

WARNING

FOOD INTOLERANCE TESTS: BUYER BEWARE

You may see food intolerance tests marketed for people with IBS, purportedly to help you identify foods that trigger symptoms such as pain and bloating. For example, immunoglobulin G (IgG) food intolerance tests involve taking a sample of your blood containing the IgG antibodies, exposing it to a variety of food items, and measuring the degree to which the IgG antibody binds to the food item. The theory is that the more binding that occurs, the more intolerant you are to the food. You then receive a report directing you to reduce or eliminate specific foods from your diet to improve symptoms.

Unfortunately, these costly tests have not been proven scientifically valid, and some professional orders and associations have actually denounced them. Food intolerances are typically determined through patterns of symptoms rather than through special testing. See a registered dietitian for guidance.

>> **Dietitian services:** The Academy of Nutrition and Dietetics website (www.eatright.org) allows you to search for registered dietitians who may have experience in GI disorders. IBS patient support groups may also be able to point you toward dietitian services in your area.

>> **Psychologists:** The American Psychological Association (APA) has an online tool that allows you to search for psychologists who may offer mind-body interventions. Just head to https://locator.apa.org. If you want to find a *gastrointestinal psychologist* (a psychologist who specializes in working with people with gastrointestinal disorders), contact a local digestive disease organization or patient support group.

If you're outside the United States, look for similar organizations in your own country.

TIP

Managing IBS in Different Environments

Part of a good quality of life is the freedom to go places and do things that interest you, without being held back by symptoms. True, not everywhere is it equally easy to maintain your equilibrium with IBS and control your symptoms. But people who have lived with IBS for a long time have come up with ways to manage the condition in all kinds of different situations, whether at home, at work, at school, in public, or in other people's homes — not to mention while eating out, while traveling, or while dating and being intimate.

Some of the best tips for each situation are detailed in this section.

Not every strategy will work for you. Try what fits with your personal situation and is likely to make a difference for you.

REMEMBER

At home

In general, many people with IBS feel the most comfortable at home because they have access to private space and everything they typically need to manage their IBS symptoms. However, here are some possible ways to increase your comfort even when you're at home:

TIP

>> **Create a feel-good aesthetic.** Consider what items you can surround yourself with that bring you joy. Do you love a clean, white space with no clutter, or would you rather see a shelf full of figurines and plants? Do you love a certain style of artwork? Try to create at least one space in your home

(even if it's one corner of a room) that's specifically designed to look good and bring you comfort.

» **Try heat therapy.** Some people find comfort in using a hot water bottle, electric heating pad, or bean- or grain-filled heating pad to soothe pain and cramping.

» **Soak in a warm bath.** You may find that a warm (not hot) bath eases stress and reduces your digestive symptoms.

» **Use aromatherapy.** A diffuser with fragrant essential oil may create a calming home environment that helps you manage your symptoms. Otherwise, try applying a skin-safe peppermint oil (typically one drop of peppermint essential oil plus three to four drops of a carrier oil) to your abdomen and massaging gently in a clockwise direction.

At work

Lost days of work are very common for people with IBS. When you're working for an employer, calling in sick may mean a loss of income, causing financial strain and uncertainty.

Work situations vary greatly, so it can be difficult to generalize about what helps make life at work easier for people with IBS. The increase in remote work, initially spurred by the COVID-19 pandemic, has undoubtedly been a relief for many people with IBS. Working from home may bring more flexibility to your day and increase your ability to deal with your symptoms in private. However, not everyone with IBS can work from home all the time.

TIP

So, what should you do in the workplace when you suspect that symptoms may strike? Here are some tips, brought to you by people living and working with IBS:

» **Meet with your manager or human resources.** Before any issues arise, try to have a friendly meeting with your manager or your employer's human resources professional (if you're comfortable doing so). In the conversation, emphasize your commitment to doing your job well and your desire to find solutions for when your symptoms flare up. You may be able to arrange for simple changes, such as working in close proximity to a restroom.

» **Manage your time.** Stress is more likely to increase when you're pressed for time in your work tasks. Try to get ahead of your deadlines and practice good time management so you avoid stressful last-minute crunches. You may even want to take shorter breaks if it allows you to complete your work at a steadier and more relaxed pace.

>> **Seek flexibility.** Identify the parts of your work that are more difficult for you to manage with your symptoms. See if you can arrange some flexibility around those particular parts of the job — for example, staggering your work hours or being able to work from home a certain number of days per week or month.

>> **Reduce stress if possible.** If you're making choices about which tasks or projects to take on, seek out the ones that are likely to be less stressful.

>> **Establish a bathroom routine.** If possible, proactively visit the bathroom at work on a set schedule. For example, you may get into a routine of going to the bathroom before every conference call to give yourself more peace of mind during the call.

>> **Dress the part.** If you can, dress in comfortable clothing with a loose waist-band to help reduce pressure on your abdomen and discomfort from your symptoms. Lots of business-appropriate clothing may be loose and comfortable.

>> **Keep moving.** Try to find ways to take movement breaks while you work. Exercising in the morning before work can help make the day more manageable. If you already have a physically active job, remember the importance of exercising outside of work for pleasure. Find a form of physical activity that's enjoyable to you and that moves your body differently from when you're at your job. For example, someone who's a mail carrier, whose job involves a lot of walking and carrying mail and packages, may benefit from yoga or Pilates.

At school

TIP

School is a unique environment that often requires in-person attendance, with someone evaluating your performance. Here are some tips for managing IBS symptoms during school:

>> **Do your accommodation homework.** Inquire in advance about any supports or accommodations you may be entitled to with a digestive health condition.

>> **Talk with your teacher or instructor.** Ask for a moment of the teacher's time and give your IBS elevator pitch (see Chapter 6) as soon as possible. That way, if any difficult situations come up, your teacher will already be aware of what you're dealing with.

THE COURTESY FLUSH: YES OR NO?

Say you're in a public restroom and you need to have a bowel movement. When your stool hits the toilet bowl, you may be worried about the smell starting to emerge. This is when you might reach behind you, while still sitting on the toilet, and perform what's called a *courtesy flush*. The courtesy flush is somewhat controversial: Some people argue it's good manners and you should practice this flushing technique at all times while in public restrooms. Others argue it's unnecessary and a big waste of water, not to mention a way to spread extra microorganisms throughout the area. And then there are the automatic flush toilets, which sometimes do the courtesy flush whether you like it or not. Just know you have the option of a courtesy flush if it seems right for you.

In public places

Many times, socializing with others means going out in public. And some people with IBS become quite nervous about going out in public for a longer period of time, especially to unfamiliar places where they may not know where and how they can access a bathroom.

TIP

For better confidence in public places, consider the following tips:

>> **Locate bathrooms.** When you're out, take a moment to find out where the nearest available bathroom is. You may be able to ask an employee of a business for special permission to use the staff toilet, or use a toilet-finder app (see "Using technology," earlier in this chapter).

>> **Time your food and drinks.** Before you go on a longer outing, try to eat only safe foods that don't trigger your symptoms, or eat lighter meals.

>> **Be prepared.** Prepare a small IBS emergency kit that fits inside a purse or backpack. This may include wet wipes, before-you-go toilet spray, peppermint candies or tea bags, medications, or perhaps a change of clothing or under-wear (see Chapter 22 for some of the essential items). There's no harm in wearing an incontinence product for extra protection if you'll be in a very uncertain situation or if you expect long lines for the bathrooms, such as when you're attending a concert or festival.

In others' homes

Spending time in other people's homes can pose unique challenges for someone with IBS. Although it's not quite as unpredictable as visiting a public place (all homes are sure to have some kind of toilet available), you'll want to adhere to the rules of etiquette and social norms, respecting your host's space.

THE MARIKO AOKI PHENOMENON

In 1985, a woman in Japan named Mariko Aoki wrote a short letter for a Japanese magazine describing a seemingly bizarre phenomenon she experienced: Whenever she was browsing in a bookstore, she felt an overwhelming need to have a bowel movement. The letter would have gone unnoticed, except that other people wrote to the magazine and said they'd experienced the same thing. The topic, in years since, has been discussed extensively online and in the media in Japan. The phenomenon turned out to be globally applicable and isn't just limited to bookstores, either: Some people experience it while shopping in clothing stores or big-box stores.

So far, science hasn't come up with a good explanation for why this happens. Possibly the relaxing activity of browsing and shopping creates the urge. Or the particular scents of the products in the stores may stimulate the olfactory nerve, which then activates the digestive tract. All in all, the phenomenon's origins remain a puzzle. But in the meantime, if you have IBS-C, don't discount the positive effects of a nice afternoon browsing at the bookstore. For best results, grab a coffee before you start browsing. (Pro tip: Be sure to locate the bookstore's restroom in advance.)

Your comfort level in someone else's space may depend on several factors: how well you know the person, the type of gathering, who else is present, and the physical layout of the dwelling. If you're visiting a close family member whose house you know well, you may be able to sneak away to the upstairs bathroom, for example, if you feel a sense of bowel urgency coming on. But if you're gathering for a baby shower in the house of someone you've never met before, you may need to handle your symptoms differently.

TIP

Here are some tips for making a visit to someone else's home go well:

>> **Visit the bathroom as soon as you arrive.** Even if you don't have to go, pay a visit to the loo so you'll know where it is later on and you don't have to potentially interrupt the host at a critical moment. If you're comfortable, you can even mention that you have a sensitive stomach — they may be able to let you know if there's another bathroom in a more discreet location.

>> **Keep the essentials close.** Slip a travel-size before-you-go toilet spray in your pocket before you leave home. That way, if the only bathroom is in close proximity to where people are gathering, you don't have to worry about smells giving you away.

>> **Be proactive about the menu.** If you're eating at someone's house, try to contact the host in advance and let them know about any dietary restrictions you have. However, don't expect the host to cater to you completely; offer to bring something that you can safely eat and share it with others.

>> **Stick to your routine during overnight visits.** If you're staying overnight at someone's house, adhere to your normal routine as much as possible. If no food is available during your regular mealtime, have a snack that you bring along and then eat lightly when the meal is served later. Remember to stay hydrated, too.

While eating out

If you have a special diet for managing your IBS, eating out can pose challenges. But with a little planning you can enjoy restaurant outings and take part in any social occasion. Here are some insider tips:

>> **Choose the establishment carefully.** Some places make it much easier to accommodate a special diet than other places. For example, some restaurants are only too happy to accommodate dietary restrictions, while other places are unable or unwilling to do so. Call in advance if you have questions about how the establishment can accommodate your diet.

>> **Check the menu in advance.** Many restaurants have menus posted online, allowing you to identify safe options or figure out what modifications to request.

>> **Ask for menu simplifications.** Opt for grilled meat, fish, or vegetable dishes without sauces or seasonings. Ask for sauces on the side, so you can control how much of them you consume.

>> **Be aware of beverages.** When dining out, limit carbonated drinks, alcohol, and caffeine, which can trigger symptoms. Stick to water or herbal teas, which are gentler on the gut.

>> **Avoid overeating.** Portion sizes can often be large in restaurants. As a result, your digestive system may be overwhelmed even by foods that don't normally trigger your symptoms. Smaller portions are key in IBS, so consider sharing a dish or taking leftovers home to avoid overeating.

While traveling

Travel tends to come with a lot of unpredictability and spontaneity. When you're on a trip, you may not know how long things will take, or exactly where and when you'll find your next meal.

If you love traveling and have IBS, don't worry — you can still experience all kinds of adventures while managing your symptoms. Here are some ways to make your travel go more smoothly:

>> **Research your location in advance.** If possible, choose a destination and accommodations that give you a variety of options for food choices. Ideally you'd have your pick of restaurants and cafés, as well as grocery or convenience stores to fill in the gaps. You may also want to check the availability and privacy of bathrooms along your journey. (For example, if you're traveling by coach bus, you may inquire whether the bus is equipped with a toilet.)

>> **Choose your travel companion wisely.** Make sure your travel partner is aware of your IBS and willing to change plans if necessary along the way.

>> **Bring your familiar medications.** If you tend to rely on over-the-counter medications to keep your symptoms under control, bring a supply from home because you may not be able to find the same type or brand at your destination. Out of caution, for international travel make sure the medication is not in a category of prohibited substances at your destination.

>> **Schedule flexible time.** Don't pack your day with too many activities when you reach your destination. Leave some time for rest and relaxation.

The good news is that many people with IBS report that their symptoms almost miraculously disappear when they're traveling or on vacation, even when eating things they don't normally eat. If you find yourself in this situation, enjoy yourself on this mini symptom-cation. See if you can implement some of the winning strategies when you get home.

During dating and intimacy

People with IBS often report that their symptoms result in decreased intimacy and/or less frequent sex. Dating, in particular, can be daunting because of the uncertainty about how a potential partner will respond when you're dealing with IBS symptoms. According to hundreds of people who've shared their dating experiences in online forums, if you're looking for a long-term relationship, the best policy is to be up-front about your IBS. Give your IBS elevator pitch (see Chapter 6) early on in the relationship. That way, if they're the type of person who has no empathy for your situation and no intention of accommodating your needs, you'll avoid wasting time going out with them again. But as one person wrote in an IBS online group: "If they're the right one, they won't care."

TIP

Here are some tips that may reduce the impact of IBS on dating and intimacy:

>> **Communicate openly (when you're comfortable doing so).** Whether you're in a new relationship or a long-standing one, communicate about how you're feeling and what you need during times when you're intimate. You don't need to go into all the details of your symptoms, but letting your partner know your needs may help them understand and help find a solution.

>> **Pay attention to timing.** If a big meal tends to trigger your symptoms, find creative date ideas that don't involve eating. Try to plan dates or intimate times when your IBS symptoms tend to be more manageable.

>> **Go slowly with intimacy.** Physical intimacy can sometimes trigger symptoms, especially if you're experiencing bloating or distension. Monitor how you feel during intimate times and let your partner know if you need a break.

Grappling with the Future

One reason living with IBS can interfere with your quality of life is that the future can feel quite unknown. You might grapple with questions such as: Will I always have the same intensity of symptoms, or will they get better or worse? How will my symptoms affect my life's goals?

Identifying and understanding your IBS triggers may give you a greater sense of control and enhance your overall quality of life. For best results, focus on maintaining a generally positive outlook by setting goals and supporting a better future for everyone living with IBS.

Setting goals

One way to make sure that IBS doesn't get in the way of your overall life path is to make sure you set goals and check in on them from time to time.

You may consider setting two types of goals:

>> Goals related to your IBS (such as reducing one specific symptom)

>> Goals for your life in general (such as gaining a skill or achieving a level of education)

Make sure you write down your goals. Keep them realistic so you can feel a sense of accomplishment and raise the bar for the next goal. Sharing your goals with a trusted friend or family member may provide additional support and encouragement to help you reach your goals.

Supporting a better future for people with IBS

A great way to stay positive about the future is to put some effort into creating a better future for everyone who lives with IBS. Incredible strides in understanding IBS have been made in the past two decades, and even more progress is expected in the years ahead as long as effort and resources continue to be spent appropriately.

TIP

Here are some ways you can support progress on IBS that may benefit you in your lifetime, as well as people who come after you:

>> **Help fundraise for IBS organizations.** Some organizations specifically fund IBS research or supports for people living with IBS. See how you can help with their fundraising efforts — for example, sharing information on social media or taking part in a charity run.

>> **Take part in a study on IBS.** You can support clinical trials for new drugs or other studies for IBS by seeing which studies are recruiting participants in your area and asking whether you're a good candidate for participation. You can also help spread the word about clinical trials even if you're not a good candidate. These actions help move studies forward, demonstrating the safety and efficacy of new medications and other treatments.

4
Coping with IBS at Specific Times

Chapter **14**

Dealing with IBS in Childhood

L oud thunderstorms, getting lost in a crowd, monsters under the bed — these are typical childhood fears. But some children fear something else altogether — debilitating abdominal pain or having to spend long hours sitting on the toilet.

Even though irritable bowel syndrome (IBS) is most frequently diagnosed in early adulthood, between 3 percent and 25 percent of children 18 and under experience symptoms that may qualify them for an IBS diagnosis. IBS can be present even in infants, where *regurgitation* (spitting up what's been swallowed) and *colic* (frequent or prolonged crying) are the most common symptoms. In toddlers and older children, constipation is the most common symptom, although children's experiences can vary widely and the symptoms may include diarrhea and urgency, intestinal gas, and nausea.

This chapter covers the risk factors for developing IBS in childhood, how IBS is diagnosed, and some practical treatment strategies for helping your child live well with IBS while minimizing its effect on their life.

Diagnosing IBS in Childhood

Abdominal pain in children is a complaint that's responsible for around 5 percent of all family doctor visits and 9 percent of pediatrician visits. IBS diagnosis in childhood uses the same criteria as in adulthood, so your child's doctor can evaluate their stomach pain relative to the criteria for IBS set out by the Rome Foundation (see Chapter 2).

IBS must be diagnosed medically and involves meeting the criteria for symptoms, as well as ruling out conditions that can manifest in a similar way. Such conditions include celiac disease and inflammatory bowel disease (IBD), as well as some disorders unique to children; the list of conditions to rule out may vary depending on the child's personal factors and medical history. To rule out these other conditions, additional tests may be required. But many medical practitioners try to strike a balance between diagnostic certainty and avoiding unnecessary invasive testing in children.

WARNING

Here are possible warning signs that something more serious than IBS may be occurring:

>> The child has close relatives with IBD, celiac disease, or peptic ulcer disease.

>> The child has persistent pain on the right side of the abdomen.

>> The child is experiencing persistent vomiting.

>> There is blood in the child's stool.

>> The child wakes up at night with diarrhea.

>> The child is experiencing unintended weight loss or slowing of growth.

The root causes of IBS in children are likely to be similar to those in adults, but most of the relevant research studies have been conducted in adults so scientists haven't yet established this with certainty.

Sometimes IBS truly emerges for the first time in adulthood, but other times people who are diagnosed in adulthood may look back and recall certain IBS-like symptoms in childhood, too — for example, long periods of time sitting on the toilet and straining to pass stool, or needing to run to the toilet urgently with diarrhea before a performance or another important event.

Some factors may pose a challenge to establishing an official medical diagnosis of IBS at a young age. For example, a child may:

>> Fail to recognize that what they're experiencing is abnormal

>> Delay letting an adult know about their symptoms

>> Believe they should tough out their symptoms

>> Feel embarrassed to discuss their symptoms

>> Have difficulty communicating clearly about their symptoms (which they may be experiencing behind a closed bathroom door)

The sidebar "Talking the talk about IBS with kids" has some tips for clear communication between all parties.

TALKING THE TALK ABOUT IBS WITH KIDS

If IBS is suspected in a child, clear communication is the foundation on which a diagnosis is built. But communicating about pain and bowel movements with children may be harder than it seems. Do you actually have to barge into the bathroom and take a look in the toilet to get at the truth? You may be able to spare yourself this unpleasant task — and spare your child the embarrassment — by following these tips for clear communication about symptoms:

- **Keep discussions calm.** Always remain calm and matter-of-fact when discussing your child's symptoms. Try not to overreact or overcompensate with humor — strong emotional reactions from you could affect your child's feelings about their own symptoms and their willingness to open up. And research shows that when children report abdominal pain, a strong emotional reaction or excessive attention from the parent can worsen the perceived pain.

- **Use books as conversation starters.** There are lots of different books on digestive health with age-appropriate language for children. For example, if constipation is suspected in a very young child, a book such as *Boo Can't Poo* by Xiao Jing "Iris" Wang, MD (Mayo Clinic Press Kids), may be helpful for giving the child an overview of what constipation means and what to do about it.

- **Follow your child's lead on language.** At first, ask open-ended questions about what they feel; then reflect their own words back to them to get more information. For example, if a child says they feel "butterflies" (their interpretation of cramping), then you can ask if the butterflies move around or stay in one place.

- **Use visual aids.** If you need to establish how frequently a symptom such as diarrhea is occurring, it may be helpful to ask the child to use a sticker chart or other visual way to record normal versus loose bowel movements.

Risk factors for pediatric IBS

Similar to adult IBS, the causes of childhood IBS are complex and dependent on personal circumstances and biology (including how sensitive the child is to pain). However, the following factors may increase a child's risk for developing IBS:

» **Adverse childhood experiences (ACEs) and other psychological factors:** ACEs are potentially traumatic events — for example, violence, abuse, or neglect — that occur in childhood. Children with more ACEs growing up are more likely to develop IBS, with a possible long-term impact on the severity of symptoms. In addition, children who currently experience anxiety, depression, or other mental health conditions may have an increased risk for IBS.

» **Age:** Some research indicates that children ages 8 to 12 have the highest rates of IBS, with decreased prevalence in children older than 12.

» **Family history of IBS:** A child is more likely to have IBS if one or both parents also have it, but so far, it's uncertain whether genes or behaviors contribute the most to this association.

» **Gut infections:** Some children develop post-infectious IBS after food poisoning or another kind of bacterial gastrointestinal infection.

» **Unhealthy eating habits:** Although food doesn't necessarily *cause* IBS, a study found that adolescents who consume fried foods and spicy foods daily had a greater risk of developing childhood IBS.

» **Low physical activity:** Children who get less physical activity and spend more time on screens may have a greater chance of developing IBS.

How IBS may impact development

Rest assured, most children with IBS grow and develop in a normal, age-appropriate manner. IBS may be uncomfortable, but it's not associated with serious complications for children's health. However, children with IBS or IBS-like symptoms often feel unwell and are shown to have a reduced quality of life. In general, IBS can be quite distressing to both a child and their parent/caregiver.

WARNING

Here are some signs that the symptoms of IBS may be having a negative impact on a child's overall well-being or relationship with food:

» Avoiding socializing or eating meals outside the home because they're afraid of symptoms

>> Frequently using over-the-counter medications to manage pain and other symptoms

>> Eating very little or avoiding foods in an attempt to control abdominal pain

>> Experiencing poor sleep quality (with a lack of proper sleep potentially worsening pain and putting a damper on mood)

For some children, even those with an IBS diagnosis, the symptoms resolve themselves within about two years. However, the majority of children will need to find ways to actively treat the disorder if they want to find relief.

Treating IBS in Childhood

As with IBS in adulthood, IBS in childhood has no cure. However, many actions may help relieve the symptoms and, therefore, decrease their impact on a child's life.

Many of the management options that work for adults, as described in Chapters 7 through 12, also apply to children. Modifications are likely needed to fit the child's routines and preferences. For medications and supplements, the doses and safety precautions may be different than they are in adults.

REMEMBER

For best results, work with your doctor to manage your child's IBS symptoms holistically through diet, environment, and other lifestyle factors. During the process of management, take the time and effort to communicate clearly and understand what your child and their doctor are saying — effective three-way communication between you, your child, and their doctor will lead to the best results.

Eating to support healthy development with IBS

How and what a child eats can help relieve IBS symptoms and support healthy development. The foundational principles of diet for children with IBS are to eat calmly and mindfully, to establish good nutrition and hydration, and to avoid foods that trigger symptoms.

Eating calmly and mindfully

TIP

Sometimes symptoms in children can be greatly reduced by establishing calming routines around mealtimes. Here are some tips for more peaceful eating patterns:

>> **Find a calm environment.** Some children have difficulty eating at school or another busy, noisy place. If possible, help your child find a quiet place to eat lunch at school, or encourage them to consume smaller, more frequent meals to manage hunger throughout the school day.

>> **Eat slowly.** Chewing each bite deliberately and taking the time to eat and enjoy the meal can go a long way toward reducing symptoms.

>> **Avoid multitasking during meals.** Put away electronic devices, books, and homework while eating.

>> **Eat together and relax at mealtimes.** A child may feel less rushed to finish a meal and less anxious if the family dines together at the table and stays until everyone finishes their meal. Dinnertime conversation is good, but make it a family rule to avoid talking while you have food in your mouth.

Another strategy is to separate solids from liquids during meals, eating only one at a time. If possible, children should wear loose-fitting clothing while eating for greater comfort.

Establishing good nutrition and hydration

To have the best chance of feeling better with IBS and maintain a positive relationship with food, children need to have a foundation of good nutrition and hydration to support their development. This can be difficult in IBS, because children may avoid many foods in an attempt to control their symptoms, leading to undesired consequences such as weight loss or, in extreme cases, nutritional deficiencies. If you notice food avoidances, it's important to ask your child why they're avoiding specific foods.

TIP

Here are the top tips for maintaining good nutrition and hydration in children with IBS:

>> **Identify triggers.** Keep a symptom and food diary (see Chapter 7) to help pinpoint problem foods.

>> **Offer a variety of foods.** Even though children may prefer the same foods time after time, offer different types of fruits, vegetables, and lean meats while limiting highly processed and fast foods.

>> **Drink up.** Encourage water between meals and limit sugary drinks and drinks with caffeine. Staying hydrated can make stools easier to pass.

>> **Find the fiber sweet spot.** Often, especially for children with constipation as their primary IBS symptom, an initial strategy is to add more fiber to the diet. Soluble fiber is often helpful, but insoluble fiber can increase gas and bloating. Encourage children to eat a wide variety of fruits (including dried fruits such as prunes) to help soften and add bulk to the stool.

>> **Watch how you talk about foods.** Avoid labeling foods as "bad," and instead focus on how each food makes them feel.

>> **Consider the role of dairy.** If your child struggles with diarrhea, a trial of a lactose-free diet may be helpful.

>> **Trial a specific probiotic.** Some probiotic strains have been shown to be helpful in alleviating abdominal pain in children. These strains include Lactobacillus GG, *Lactobacillus reuteri* DSM 17938, and *Bacillus coagulans* LactoSpore (Align). Generally, it can be helpful to have your child try the probiotic for four weeks to see if their abdominal pain improves.

To manage IBS, children should also avoid specific foods that trigger symptoms. The process of finding food triggers for IBS symptoms is the same in kids as it is in adults (see Chapter 7).

Like adults, children with IBS sometimes benefit from adopting a low-FODMAP diet (described in Chapter 8). Research on the low-FODMAP diet specifically in children is still emerging, and this diet in a child or teen should be implemented under the guidance of a registered dietitian. Because children and teens are still growing and developing, their nutrition needs are different than those of adults and they need to be monitored closely. Because of the restrictive nature of the diet, it's also important that mealtimes are still enjoyed and a positive relationship with food is maintained.

Other treatment strategies for children with IBS

In addition to changing how and what a child eats, several other treatment strategies exist for IBS in children. These include bathroom routines, mental health and ACE management, exercise, and sometimes medications.

Bathroom routines

Establishing a regular bathroom routine for bowel movements can be helpful for children, increasing predictability and helping reduce symptoms. Although a child with constipation may want to minimize time on the toilet, they can be encouraged to relax and sit for a predetermined amount of time to focus on the task at hand. A toilet stool (see Chapter 12) may also be useful for establishing a good toilet posture.

Mental health management

When a child has IBS, stress or uncertainty may be a frequent trigger of symptoms — understandably, because stress has known effects on gut functioning. Situations such as a test at school or family problems can be stressful for many kids and may be associated with symptoms.

REMEMBER

Stress is a personal, internal experience. A situation that's not very stressful for one person may be very stressful for another. So, if you see that something appears stressful for a child with IBS, take care to manage it, regardless of how *you* feel about it yourself.

TIP

Here are some ways to help children reduce stress:

>> **Provide a listening ear.** Give the child opportunities to talk about their worries with a trusted adult or friend, but don't pressure them to open up.

>> **Celebrate effort.** Praise a child's effort rather than their achievement. For example, say "I'm impressed with your dedication to studying for that test" instead of commenting on their final score (even if they do well).

>> **Aim for a calm and predictable schedule.** Adjusting a child's weekly routine to provide more predictability, and not trying to cram too much into each day, may help the child feel more secure and reduce stress.

>> **Manage caregiver stress.** Learn to manage your own stress. If you appear angry or upset, your child may have more difficulty staying calm.

In addition, children may benefit from mind-body interventions such as the following (see Chapter 11 for more information):

>> Gut-directed hypnotherapy

>> Cognitive behavioral therapy (CBT)

>> Breathing techniques

>> Mindfulness and meditation

>> Yoga

Evidence exists for the benefits of these therapies, although more needs to be known about how they work in children specifically.

ACE management

Managing the effects of ACEs is a lifelong endeavor and is especially important for children with IBS. In addition to the general strategies for mental health management, ACE management may include the following:

>> **Find a counselor.** A qualified therapist specializing in pediatrics may help a child process their experiences and cope more effectively.

>> **Show affection.** With both your actions and your words, show the child you care on a regular basis. With that said, ask for permission before you show physical gestures of affection such as hugging.

>> **Encourage connections with a safe, trusted adult.** Children become more resilient and secure when they have support from a trusted adult such as a teacher, coach, or family friend who cares about their well-being.

Exercise

Staying active may be another great way to reduce the impact of IBS in a child's life. Although few studies have been done specifically in children, children with IBS benefit from fun, moderate-intensity activities such as:

>> Running and playing outside (in a safe area, such as a park or playground)

>> Riding bicycles with a friend or family member

>> Hiking on a short nature trail

>> Walking a dog

>> Dancing

REMEMBER

During activities, pay attention to any signs that your child's IBS symptoms are interfering with the fun. Take a break from the activity if symptoms seem to intensify or if the child experiences a feeling of bowel urgency. Communicate that staying active keeps them healthy, and it's also okay to take a break when needed.

Medicines

If other types of treatments don't manage to get your child's IBS symptoms under control, a doctor may prescribe medications to help reduce IBS symptoms such as constipation and diarrhea (or urgency). Some of the medications or supplements available for adults are also used in children, but they may have special warnings, so always follow the dose and timing recommended by your doctor.

REMEMBER

Note that all supplements and over-the-counter medications should be cleared with your doctor before you give them to a child. For example, when a child has constipation, laxatives that you buy at a drugstore should be used with caution because kids can become reliant on them over time and the products may lead to electrolyte abnormalities and dehydration.

JULIA'S CASE: DIETARY CHANGE TO SUPPORT GUT HEALTH

Julia is a 13-year-old competitive dancer who struggles with IBS symptoms, including abdominal pain, bloating, and unpredictable diarrhea, which often disrupt her rehearsals and performances. Her busy and tiring schedule led to frequent meals on the go, often with processed foods, fast foods, and sugary drinks. Her symptoms started about six months ago with no clear trigger, and she recently visited her doctor and received an IBS diagnosis. Julia's mother has IBS, too.

Julia and her family met with a dietitian, who suggested a tailored dietary plan to manage her symptoms. Instead of processed foods and fast foods, Julia's meals were replaced with healthier portable options such as wraps with lean protein and fresh veggies, or yogurt with blueberries. Prepacked snacks, such as rice cakes, bananas, and nuts, were included to fuel her long practice sessions. Hydration with water and herbal teas replaced sodas, and smaller, more frequent meals were planned to avoid digestive discomfort. Additionally, Julia was guided to practice mindful eating by avoiding rushed meals (sitting down in a quiet place) and chewing slowly to support digestion. Within three months, Julia reported significant symptom relief and improved energy levels, demonstrating that even with a demanding lifestyle, dietary adjustments can effectively help manage IBS in children.

IN THIS CHAPTER

» **Being proactive in preparing for pregnancy when you have IBS**

» **Discovering how your IBS symptoms may change during pregnancy and what you can do to help keep them under control**

» **Making the birth and postpartum periods easier when you have IBS**

Chapter **15**

Handling IBS in Pregnancy

I f you have irritable bowel syndrome (IBS), you may be used to having a cute little belly bump from bloating and distension. But people with IBS who become pregnant will have a new kind of belly bump — one with a real, growing fetus inside.

When someone is pregnant, not only are the fetal cells multiplying and developing in a tightly choreographed manner within the uterus, but the pregnant person's body is adapting to the increasing demands of the fetus by increasing blood volume, expanding the kidneys, increasing oxygen consumption via the lungs, spiking levels of certain hormones, and more.

Through all these changes, the abdominal region is a crowded and busy place. Constipation is common in pregnancy as a result of hormonal changes. As the fetus grows, it may push against the digestive organs and put pressure on a gut that may already be sensitive. People with IBS report that symptoms may be affected in different ways during pregnancy:

» The symptoms can get milder or disappear altogether.

» The symptoms can get worse or harder to manage overall.

» IBS-like symptoms can emerge for the first time in pregnancy.

Because everyone is slightly different, no one can predict in advance which way your IBS will go during pregnancy. However, this chapter gives some commonly reported experiences.

REMEMBER

Here's the good news: Because IBS so often affects women of childbearing age, being pregnant with IBS is not uncommon. One small study found that around 25 percent of pregnant women had IBS. No matter how your symptoms are affected on a personal level, know that the vast majority of people with IBS have successful pregnancies that result in healthy babies. If you commit to taking care of yourself and managing your symptoms appropriately, there's a good chance you'll power right through your pregnancy until the time comes to meet your bundle of joy.

This chapter is all about what to expect when you're expecting with IBS. It covers prepregnancy planning, what pregnancy with IBS can look like, and how to manage your diet and other important aspects of your lifestyle when you're pregnant. Finally, this chapter includes some tips on handling the birth and postpartum periods when you have IBS.

One important thing to note as you read this chapter is that scientific research on IBS and pregnancy is very scarce. Scientists really need to start filling this research gap, especially given how commonly IBS is diagnosed in younger women, some of whom may aim to be pregnant. But in the meantime, the recommendations and tips in this chapter are primarily based on clinical observations and the reports of people with IBS who have been pregnant.

Planning for Pregnancy

If you have the luxury of planning in advance for your pregnancy, you can take a few actions to increase the chances that everything will go smoothly after you have a positive pregnancy test in hand.

First on the list, if you have IBS-like symptoms, is to get an accurate and official medical diagnosis of IBS. An IBS diagnosis is very important because some conditions that can affect pregnancy, such as pelvic inflammatory disease, have similar symptoms to IBS and should be ruled out. (See Chapter 5 for pointers on seeking a diagnosis.)

A common question about planning for pregnancy when you have IBS is whether IBS reduces the chances that you'll become pregnant. As far as researchers know, IBS itself does not interfere with fertility. However, your symptoms may indirectly affect your opportunities to become pregnant, for example, by reducing your libido or causing discomfort during intercourse, leading to less frequent intercourse and potentially limiting your chances for conception.

TECHNICAL STUFF

A healthy pregnancy is very likely in IBS, but some studies have found that people with IBS may have a slightly higher chance of *miscarriage* (spontaneous loss of a fetus in the first half of gestation) and *ectopic pregnancy* (in which a fertilized egg implants outside the uterus, usually in one of the fallopian tubes) than people without IBS do. However, more research is needed to verify these observations because other factors besides IBS itself could account for the findings.

If you've been diagnosed with IBS and you're planning for pregnancy, your number-one job is to make sure your symptoms are as controlled as possible before you conceive. Any test runs with medications, dietary shifts, or lifestyle changes should be explored before you try to get pregnant because you'll be better off if your IBS is in a stable state before pregnancy. Having no symptoms may not be totally achievable, but you should explore the available treatments so your symptoms are as predictable and controlled as possible. That way, you'll be better equipped to tell how the pregnancy itself is affecting you.

TIP

If you're planning to get pregnant, a preconception appointment with your doctor is a good idea. If you have IBS, this appointment is a great opportunity to ask any questions you may have about your gut symptoms in relation to pregnancy. In addition, you may want to discuss the following:

>> **If you're on medications (for IBS or otherwise), discuss whether they're safe to continue in the preconception phase or during pregnancy, and if not, what alternatives exist for keeping a handle on your symptoms.** Some medications that work well for IBS symptoms (for example, hyoscine butylbromide for abdominal pain) haven't been tested much in pregnant people, so you should discuss the available safety information with your doctor. In some cases, you may decide to switch to a nonpharmaceutical treatment alternative and give it a trial run before becoming pregnant.

>> **Let your doctor know if you're on a restrictive or elimination diet.** If you've adopted a special diet to manage your IBS symptoms, find out what nutrition supports may be available to you during pregnancy. Women often find that during pregnancy (particularly in the first trimester when loss of appetite and food aversions are common), their diet restrictions increase, so support from a registered dietitian helps ensure that they can meet their nutritional needs and avoid fetal complications while keeping symptoms under control.

REMEMBER

Generally, doctors recommend taking a daily prenatal multivitamin with 0.4 mg of folic acid before and during pregnancy.

Also remember that if you're planning to become pregnant, it's best to avoid alcohol.

Dealing with IBS While Pregnant

Seeing those double lines (or plus sign) on the pregnancy test device is the key that unlocks a whole new adventure — one that's sure to have its ups and downs but that can ultimately give you a whole new appreciation for your body's amazing capabilities.

After confirming you're pregnant, the most important thing to know is that IBS does not harm your baby. Even if you experience diarrhea as part of your IBS, you're still absorbing your food properly and will be able to nourish yourself and the fetus. Nor will you pass IBS on to your child through your genes.

REMEMBER

With that said, a few cautions are warranted when you're pregnant and have IBS:

>> **Proper nutrition and hydration are essential for a healthy pregnancy, and managing your IBS symptoms may create barriers to this.** Build time into your schedule to care for yourself, including shopping for and cooking nutritious meals. Carry water with you at all times, and plan for more bathroom breaks as you increase your hydration. Overall, eat a variety of foods and try to minimize the restrictions you put on your diet.

>> **If you experience prolonged diarrhea with no breaks you may become dehydrated.** Be sure to drink lots of water and other fluids if this happens.

WARNING

During the first trimester, nausea and vomiting are common. However, pregnant people should seek medical attention if they experience the following gastrointestinal symptoms:

>> Excessive or constant vomiting, leading to limited nutrition or trouble keeping fluids down

>> Weight loss after the first trimester of pregnancy

>> Severe abdominal pain

Knowing how your symptoms will change in pregnancy

Whether or not you have IBS, pregnancy is associated with changes in gastrointestinal functioning that may be related to the following factors:

>> The changes in hormone levels that occur in pregnancy can affect your bowel movements. For example, high levels of progesterone slow down *motility* (the way food and fluids move through your digestive tract), making constipation worse.

>> The pelvic floor changes to make room for the growing fetus, causing increased abdominal pressure that can affect your bowel movements.

>> If you're advised to take certain medications or supplements for your health in pregnancy, you may experience gastrointestinal side effects. For example, both iron to support extra blood volume in pregnancy and magnesium sulfate to treat preeclampsia or premature labor can trigger or worsen diarrhea.

Knowing how your regular IBS symptoms will change during pregnancy is a bit like spinning a prize wheel: The result can't be predicted in advance. Symptoms can go in any direction during pregnancy; they may become milder or go away, or they may stay the same or get worse. However, based on anecdotal reports of women with IBS, some general patterns may exist. Many women with IBS-D (diarrhea) say their symptoms improved during pregnancy, and women with IBS-C (constipation) say their symptoms became more difficult. Consider these typical comments from pregnant women in online chats:

> "I have IBS-D, and pregnancy really improved my symptoms a lot. I had some problems in the first trimester still, but nothing from the second trimester until birth. It was actually so nice not having to worry about that for months."

> "I have IBS-C. . . . All my usual trigger foods are so much worse on my stomach. My severe constipation is now exponentially worse."

A few lucky women even report that pregnancy had a lasting positive effect on their IBS, so both during pregnancy and after giving birth, their IBS symptoms were reduced. Some report that their IBS abdominal pain was never as severe after experiencing pregnancy.

Some people also report that IBS-like symptoms appear for the first time during pregnancy. If this happens to you, discuss the new symptoms with your doctor in case further investigation is needed. However, you may not receive a diagnosis of IBS right away because of the difficulty distinguishing the temporary effects of pregnancy from the longer-lasting symptoms of IBS. Talk with your doctor about how to safely treat the symptoms you're experiencing in pregnancy. Then, if the symptoms persist for more than three to six months after giving birth, make an appointment with your doctor to explore whether an IBS diagnosis is appropriate.

Adjusting your lifestyle habits in pregnancy

If you read the pregnancy advice books, you may notice an emphasis on changing some of your daily habits to ensure the best pregnancy outcomes. Everyone who's pregnant should put the following actions at the top of their priority list:

>> **Aim to get seven to nine hours of restful sleep every night.** Turn to Chapter 12 for tips on improving the quality and quantity of your sleep.

>> **During your waking hours, build some flexibility into your schedule so you can sit and rest when you feel the need.**

>> **Pay extra attention to your oral hygiene during pregnancy, brushing your teeth after every meal.** People who are pregnant are more vulnerable to gum inflammation and bleeding.

>> **Get some exercise every day.** In total, you should be getting around 150 minutes of moderate-intensity exercise per week, unless advised otherwise by your doctor. Swimming and brisk walking are both excellent ways to stay active during pregnancy. Just remember, pregnancy is not the time to try out a new sport or engage in higher-intensity exercise than you were doing before you got pregnant.

In addition to these baseline habits, when you have IBS it's especially important to calm the ongoing communication between your gut and your brain. Keeping your body and mind relaxed is important, both for good pregnancy outcomes and for keeping your symptoms under control. Here are some tips for keeping a handle on stress and anxiety during pregnancy:

>> Regularly engage in calming activities such as meditation or prenatal yoga. These activities can help relax both the body and the mind, helping you focus on the present moment without worry.

>> When stresses inevitably come up, try to step away and do some breathing exercises (see Chapter 11 for an example) or have a brief chat with a trusted friend for support.

>> Practice keeping your thoughts positive by doing activities you enjoy and spending time with optimistic people. You may also want to avoid movies and other media that have scary or negative themes.

Medication is another important consideration for ensuring a smooth pregnancy when you have IBS. Depending on your preference, you may decide to control new symptoms that emerge using medications or supplements that are safe during pregnancy. Here are some tips for managing your medications and supplements:

» If you want to take an over-the-counter product such as a fiber supplement with laxative effects, make sure you let the pharmacist know you're pregnant and ask for a recommendation. Otherwise, see your doctor to discuss treatment options.

» Read the labels of any over-the-counter medications you take. Make sure you're okay with the possible side effects, and double-check with your doctor that they're safe and that your dose is appropriate during pregnancy.

Optimizing your diet in pregnancy

Regardless of whether you have IBS, you should implement a few dietary changes as soon as possible when you find out you're pregnant:

» Cut out alcohol, which may harm fetal development.

» Avoid foods that have a higher chance of containing harmful microorganisms, including raw milk, soft and unpasteurized cheeses, raw fish (as in sushi), raw sprouts, raw meat and eggs, and deli and processed meats.

» Avoid eating fish with high mercury levels, such as tuna and swordfish.

» Reduce caffeine consumption, preferably below 300 mg a day — the equivalent of about two 8-ounce (250 mL) cups of coffee. Remember that caffeine can be found in other foods and drinks, and your daily total should include *all* sources of caffeine: coffee, tea (including black, oolong, white, and green tea), caffeinated soft drinks (for example, cola beverages) and energy drinks, chocolate, and herbs such as guarana and yerba mate.

» Avoid certain kinds of herbal teas that are not advisable to drink when pregnant: aloe, buckthorn bark, chamomile, coltsfoot, comfrey, duck root, juniper berry, labrador tea, lobelia, pennyroyal, sassafras, senna leaves, and stinging nettle. Other herbal teas, such as citrus peel, ginger, orange peel, and rose hip, are considered safe in moderation (two to three cups per day). Also, avoid drinking kombucha tea because of its alcohol and caffeine content, as well as its high acidity.

» Only consume fruits and vegetables that you know are washed thoroughly.

Eating for two doesn't mean eating double portions, but your nutritional requirements do increase in pregnancy, particularly during the second and third trimesters. The calories you need change during different pregnancy stages. For women with a normal-range weight before pregnancy, the recommended calorie intake beyond your usual diet is as follows:

>> **First trimester (first 12 weeks):** No additional calories needed.

>> **Second trimester (13 to 26 weeks):** Around 340 extra calories per day.

>> **Third trimester (after 26 weeks):** Around 450 extra calories per day.

To meet your nutritional needs, healthcare professionals recommend a balanced diet that includes:

>> A variety of vegetables — dark leafy greens, red and orange vegetables, legumes (beans and peas), starchy vegetables, and others

>> Fruits (especially whole fruits)

>> Grains, with an emphasis on whole grains

>> Pasteurized dairy products, including milk, yogurt, and cheese; or fortified plant-based beverages (such as soy or rice milk)

>> A variety of proteins, including seafood, lean meats and poultry, eggs, nuts, seeds, and soy products

FILLING YOUR FOLIC ACID NEEDS

Folic acid, a type of B vitamin, is present in many vitamin supplements. In foods, the same vitamin is known as folate. This vitamin is crucial for creating healthy new cells, so it's critically important in pregnancy. During early pregnancy, folic acid supports the development of the baby's spine and brain. Additionally, folic acid contributes to healthier hair, skin, and nails. Women who don't consume sufficient folic acid are at an increased risk of having a baby with neural tube defects, which are birth defects affecting the spine and brain.

Which foods are high in folate? Dark green vegetables, beans, peas, lentils, oranges, and fortified grain products are all good sources of this vitamin. However, most women don't get enough folate from food, so a supplement is almost universally recommended. Prenatal vitamins tend to have a sufficient amount.

If new gastrointestinal symptoms crop up during pregnancy and they seem to be related to what you eat, start keeping a food diary (see Chapter 7) so you can begin to identify what may be triggering the symptoms. Many women report that their food sensitivities change during pregnancy, so either they can tolerate foods they previously weren't able to tolerate, or they become sensitive to foods they previously could tolerate. If the list of foods you can't tolerate becomes extensive, or if all foods seem to make your symptoms worse, seek out the advice of a registered dietitian on how to stay well nourished.

Prepregnancy if you were keeping your IBS symptoms under control with a diet that restricts certain categories of foods, you should consult a registered dietitian after you find out you're pregnant to make sure you can meet all your nutritional needs. For example, if you were already on a diet that was effective for calming your symptoms before pregnancy, then during pregnancy you should ask a dietitian whether any food reintroductions are necessary for achieving balanced nutrition to support the growing fetus. Scientists don't yet know a lot about how the low-FODMAP diet affects pregnancy outcomes, so it's best not to start a low-FODMAP diet for the first time during pregnancy.

TECHNICAL
STUFF

FODMAP stands for *fermentable oligosaccharides, disaccharides, monosaccharides and polyols.* Read more about a low-FODMAP diet in Chapter 8.

TIP

Here are some tips for meeting your nutrition and hydration needs when you're pregnant and have IBS:

>> Try to make as many of your meals at home as you can, focusing on using a variety of fresh ingredients (and being sure to wash your fruits and vegetables well, even if the package says they're prewashed).

>> Avoid fatty and spicy foods as much as possible. If you're really craving this type of food, try a small portion.

>> Where possible, avoid ice-cold water or very cold foods because of their negative effects on gut motility.

>> Get as much fiber in your diet as you can tolerate. Whole grains, as well as fruits and vegetables, should be the mainstays of your diet, especially if your symptoms include constipation.

>> Instead of eating big meals, consume smaller and more frequent meals throughout the day. Remember to eat a variety of foods at each sitting, even when your portions are small. Try smoothies as a digestion-friendly way to consume more fruits and vegetables.

>> Carry a water bottle with you and sip water continually throughout the day. Unsweetened, unflavored carbonated water may also work, as long as it doesn't trigger additional symptoms.

Navigating Birth and the Postpartum Period with IBS

Before giving birth, most pregnant individuals put together a birth plan in consultation with their healthcare team. But if there's one thing to remember about labor and birth, it's to expect the unexpected. When you have IBS, you may feel even more uncertainty: How will you be able to distinguish between normal abdominal pain and labor pain? What if your symptoms flare up at a crucial moment in the birth process? If your labor goes on for many hours, what will you be able to eat or drink?

Before giving birth, write down your questions and concerns about the process and discuss them with your doctor, midwife, or another experienced birth professional such as a doula. You may be able to prepare for some eventual scenarios — for example, you can plan to have a variety of snacks on hand that will keep you fueled without triggering your symptoms. Overall, though, remember that the birth process may require a lot of flexibility and quick thinking.

After a successful birth, the challenge becomes finding the time to take care of yourself (and your IBS symptoms) while caring for the baby. During this time, you can be guided by the airplane safety briefings that tell you to put on your own oxygen mask before assisting someone else: Taking care of your own basic needs will make you a better caregiver.

TIP

Here are some tips for balancing out your own needs with the baby's needs in the first few weeks postpartum:

» **If possible, ask a partner or someone else you trust to stay with you for the first few days.** You should choose a helpful and nonjudgmental person who's willing to pitch in with whatever you need as you get used to life with a baby. This may help reduce your stress, which can help keep your IBS symptoms under control.

» **If you're spending time at home alone with the baby, make sure you have a safe place to put your little one for a few minutes while you take care of your own needs, such as when you go to the bathroom.** Don't worry if the baby cries for a few minutes while you do what you need to do; what matters is that the baby is safe. When you've finished taking care of your needs, you can give your full attention to comforting the baby.

» **Write down five to ten nourishing, easy-to-prepare, portable snacks and put the list in a visible location such as on the fridge.** Not only will the list give you a quick idea of what to eat when you're too exhausted to plan a meal, but it can also serve as a guide for what to buy when you go grocery shopping.

Make sure each snack has a source of protein, as well as some fiber that you can tolerate. Some examples for this list are:

- Trail mix and a mandarin orange
- Yogurt with granola
- A cut-up hard-boiled egg with hummus and whole-grain crackers

MISSION: HYDRATION

Hydration is very important for successful breastfeeding. A rule of thumb is to drink one glass of water each time you breastfeed. Drink when you're thirsty too, of course, and drink more if your urine appears dark yellow.

What should you drink? Go easy on beverages that contain artificial sweeteners and colors. Water is your best option, and adding lemon, lime, or berries can naturally infuse flavor into your water to provide some variety. If you're thinking of consuming an electrolyte solution while breastfeeding, run it by your doctor first to ensure it doesn't contain compounds that could be harmful.

Remember, too, that you can stay hydrated by eating fruits and vegetables such as melons, strawberries, lettuce, and cucumbers, which have a high water content and can increase your fluid intake while providing added nourishment.

Chapter 16

Dealing with IBS as an Athlete

It's marathon day. Hundreds of runners are lined up at the starting line in the minutes before the race. The athletes are stretching, jumping up and down, or adjusting the settings on their smartwatches. When the starter pistol fires, they're off and running. Some of the runners settle into a comfortable pace along the race route. But a few of them veer off the course right away, heading straight for the nearest restroom.

Bowel urgency is a common problem at almost every high-level athletic event. Hang around a group of elite athletes long enough, and you're likely to hear a story about going to extreme measures to find a place to go, or even losing control of the bowels altogether. Among marathoners, the affliction is sometimes called "runner's trots."

Studies show that digestive problems are common in athletes — people who push themselves to high levels of athletic performance — before, during, and after exercise. Depending on the sport, between one-third and one-half of athletes report experiencing gastrointestinal (GI) symptoms during exercise. The most common symptoms reported are abdominal pain, bowel urgency, and diarrhea. One large study on a marathon in Seaside, Oregon, reported that 18 percent of marathon runners had interrupted a race for a bowel movement. Some reported losing control of their bowels while running. Women athletes tend to experience these symptoms more often than men, and younger athletes more often than older. The GI issues during exercise may be compounded when an athlete has irritable bowel syndrome (IBS).

This chapter clarifies the relationship between high athletic performance and gut symptoms. It outlines some signs that an athlete's gut symptoms may indicate IBS rather than normal exercise-induced stress. Finally, the chapter goes over some ways to manage IBS as an athlete, including dietary changes that may help keep gut symptoms under control.

Athletic Performance and Gut Symptoms

High athletic performance puts stress on the body, causing GI symptoms even for normal, healthy athletes. Here are some of the underlying causes of exercise-induced gut symptoms:

>> Physical jostling of the GI tract, typical of high-impact exercise such as running, which may cause slower gastric emptying and other digestive disruptions.

>> Increased blood flow to the extremities during physical activity, with less blood flow to the GI tract, causing possible injury to the *epithelial* (inner) layer of the gut and an increase in gut barrier permeability; in turn, this may lead to low-level inflammation in the intestine.

>> Release of *norepinephrine* (a stress hormone) from nerve endings, which signals to the sympathetic nervous system, limiting optimal gut motility and impairing the ability to absorb nutrients.

>> Changes to the gut microbial community, which can affect gut motility and other aspects of gut function.

WARNING

When increased blood flow to your extremities and release of norepinephrine occur together, blood is diverted away from the intestine, and you're said to have *subclinical intestinal ischemia*. Normally it resolves when you stop exercising. However, in rare cases, if the reduced blood flow continues, you may develop *ischemic gut* (damage to the intestine from inadequate blood supply), characterized by abdominal pain or cramping and sometimes blood in the stool. If this happens, you should seek medical help immediately.

The contributors to exercise-induced gut symptoms can look very similar to the triggers for IBS symptoms:

>> Dehydration

>> Not consuming food or drink for an extended period of time

>> Eating certain foods — high-fat foods, high-fiber foods, spicy foods, sugar alcohols, and sometimes protein supplements — before exercising

>> Stress or excitement (commonly experienced before or during a competition)

In turn, gut symptoms often affect athletic performance. Pain and bowel urgency can affect your training regimen or even your desire to train, for example. And running to the bathroom during a competition can add critical minutes to an athlete's race time. Even athletic clothing choices can be affected when bloating or distension are at play, with snug-fitting outfits causing more discomfort.

Knowing When to Explore an IBS Diagnosis

Extreme exercise is known to induce gut symptoms, but only a small number of athletes may actually have an IBS diagnosis. One 2019 study in the United States found that IBS was underdiagnosed in athletes: Around 3 percent of endurance athletes were medically diagnosed with IBS, while around 10 percent seemingly met the criteria for IBS. Less than half had consulted a medical professional for help.

If gut symptoms are extremely common among athletes, when do they cross the line from normal digestive distress to a chronic problem that requires a diagnosis? Athletes may become accustomed to gut symptoms and think of them as a normal part of life — and exercise-induced and IBS-related gut symptoms have similar triggers. But here are some ways to tell that symptoms are going beyond what's normal for an athlete and that you should explore an IBS diagnosis:

>> Symptoms are present even after light training or on non-training days.

>> Certain foods or beverages seem to trigger symptoms regardless of exercise (although food triggers alone don't mean you have IBS).

>> You have existing anxiety, depression, or another mental health diagnosis.

>> You experience high levels of stress, unrelated to athletic competition.

>> You have a tendency toward hypervigilance (alertness and sensitivity that's hard to turn off).

Diagnosis of IBS in athletes is the same as in nonathletes but may be slightly complicated by the influence of extreme exercise during the process. Be sure to let your doctor know how your training schedule seems to relate to your pattern of bowel movements.

Considering IBS Management in Athletes

IBS in athletes is managed in largely the same way as it is in nonathletes. However, for athletes who continue to strive for high levels of performance, adaptations may help mitigate some of the gut symptoms. One main consideration is that moderate forms of exercise appear beneficial for managing gut symptoms (see Chapter 12), whereas high-intensity or long-duration exercise are associated with more gut symptoms overall. A 2021 study in Canada found that people with IBS experience more symptoms after exercise than athletes without IBS, with the most common symptoms being pain or cramps, bloating, and diarrhea.

TIP

Some special adaptations may be necessary, but it's very possible for people with an IBS diagnosis to achieve high athletic performance. Here are some tips for managing IBS symptoms as an athlete:

>> **Develop a routine for bowel movements.** Try to develop a bowel movement habit at a certain time each day. Fit your training schedule around it so you're less likely to be struck by bowel urgency during exercise.

>> **Listen to your body.** Figure out how long or fast you can train without inducing gut symptoms, and try to work around those limits. Or if you're training and you suddenly feel bowel urgency coming on, be prepared to adjust your plan.

>> **Use yoga as a way to cross-train.** Take a yoga class when you're not training for your main sport. You'll improve your mind-body communication and reduce stress. You may also pick up a breathing exercise that helps you manage pre-competition stress (see the sidebar "Breathing right for a fight").

>> **Journal about your athletic performance.** Either on paper or digitally, jot down a few points about your diet, athletic performance, and symptoms each day. See if you can identify any patterns.

>> **Reduce stress during training.** To reduce your nervous energy, try to focus on your enjoyment of the sport rather than on measurements of performance.

Despite all these pointers, you may find it's inevitable that you'll deal with increased gut symptoms as you train harder, so you need to plan accordingly, with bathroom stops along your route or looser clothing while you train. Modify your activity as needed to make symptoms more manageable.

BREATHING RIGHT FOR A FIGHT

The day had come for the North American Karate Championships. Two months previously, author Maitreyi had just won the Karate Canada 2009 National Championships and was coming off a performance high. Now at the North American event, the competition would be stiffer than ever. She had been unable to sleep the night before, all-consumed by the excitement and pressure of performance. She intentionally got up early on the morning of the competition to fuel with bananas, peanut butter and rye toast, instant breakfast mix, and scrambled eggs. This large breakfast was very different from her usual habit of consuming coffee and fruit, but knowing the competition flow of the day, she was aware that if she performed well, she wouldn't have another opportunity to eat until at least 9 o'clock that night. However, consuming the food wasn't easy because she had no appetite, and her nerves were at an all-time high. (From medical school and onward in high-pressure situations, Maitreyi's gut would bear the brunt of stress — classic situational IBS — at least until she became a student of yoga in 2016.) Then the competition began. Her first two matches went well, as she progressed into the final round. At this point, she faced the previous Pan American Champion and knew she would need to bring everything she had to the fight. Somehow, she remembered an activated breathing exercise that the national coach had taught the team months before. Although she hadn't practiced it regularly (although she wished she had), somehow it flowed effortlessly when she started employing it. Maitreyi closed her eyes, sat with an erect spine in a corner, practiced her breathing exercise for less than a minute, and visualized the outcome she wanted. After this exercise, she was completely energized — and she literally had the fight of her life.

Nourishing Your Body as an Athlete with IBS

Athletes have a high requirement for energy intake. As an athlete with IBS, the timing of meals and the items you eat and drink can have a significant impact on your gut symptoms. One study found that athletes with IBS tended to more carefully manage their food choices to control their symptoms, resulting in a more restricted diet than other athletes. However, achieving a baseline of good nutrition and hydration is important as well, to optimize your performance as an athlete.

TIP

The diet that works best for you will depend on your sport, as well as personal factors and preferences. Here are some guidelines for good nutrition and hydration as an athlete with IBS:

» Pay attention to hydration even when you're not exercising, and start every training session well-hydrated. Sip on fluids (water, as well as sports drinks if you can tolerate them) regularly throughout the day.

» Reduce consumption of alcohol, which can generally irritate the gut and cause digestive symptoms.

» Eat plenty of high-fiber foods on a regular basis. Choose complex carbohydrates and minimize simple sugars.

» Avoid eating large meals; instead, consume smaller amounts of food throughout the day, whether on rest days or training days.

REMEMBER

Don't hesitate to see a specialist sports dietitian with knowledge of IBS if you want specific advice about which foods to eat to meet your nutritional needs.

Beyond what an athlete eats on a regular basis, their pre-sport meal may have some special significance for how they perform. Athletes typically pay attention to what they eat in two periods of time before training or competing:

» Several hours (two to three) before engaging in training or competition, complex carbohydrates are recommended because they burn slowly, allowing for a constant glucose supply to fuel your performance. During this time, avoid high-fat, high-fiber foods. Good choices include bananas, nuts, or oatmeal. Meanwhile, be sure to drink lots of hydrating fluids leading up to the start of exercise.

» Right before exercising, typically athletes carbo-load, or eat foods such as bagels or pasta that are largely composed of simple (quick-burning) carbohydrates to give immediate energy. For some athletes with IBS, these foods may trigger symptoms. Gentle-on-the-stomach alternatives, to try are rice cakes with peanut butter, gluten-free oatmeal with banana, or plain white rice or sweet potatoes.

Experiment with the timing of your eating patterns. You may even decide to extend your pre-competition way of eating to several days before the competition for best results.

TIP

With IBS, in addition to basic nutritional advice, the goal is also to avoid triggering symptoms through gut-irritating foods. Here are some tips for your pre-competition period as an athlete with IBS:

>> If you know you're sensitive to FODMAPs, avoid high-FODMAP foods, including dairy products, gluten, and high-FODMAP fruits such as apples and pears.

TECHNICAL STUFF

FODMAP stands for fermentable oligosaccharides, disaccharides, monosaccharides and polyols. Read more about a low-FODMAP diet in Chapter 8.

>> If you've previously, had symptoms (cramps or abdominal pain during exercise) from high-fiber foods such as legumes, avoid them.

>> Avoid coffee, tea, and other caffeine-containing beverages, which can increase gut motility and thereby create the urge for a bowel movement.

>> Try not to consume foods you've never tried before.

>> Don't compete without having eaten in the past few hours.

>> Don't eat a large meal before a competition; instead, increase your carbohydrate intake in the days leading up to the race with small, frequent meals.

BARS AND GELS AND CHEWS, OH MY

During long training sessions or races, athletes need to maintain their energy by consuming sports drinks or various foods. Many products exist for this purpose — energy bars, gels, and chews. However, you may need to be cautious about which ones you consume, because many of them contain gut-irritating ingredients that can worsen diarrhea. Sugar alcohols are a common ingredient that can increase gut symptoms, and some products contain caffeine. Make sure you consume drinks specially formulated for endurance athletes, because sweet drinks such as juices without balanced electrolytes may make you feel worse. For endurance athletes, products formulated with lower sugar content or natural sweeteners may support electrolyte balance. Finding the products and brands that work best for you may take some trial and error. But when you find them, make sure you stick to them during a race so a new brand of gel doesn't suddenly send you running to the nearest restroom.

5

Eating Well with IBS

Find valuable practical tips for successfully managing your symptoms through what you eat.

Put into practice your knowledge about dietary management of IBS by creating meals and snacks that may reduce your symptoms.

Make tasty, IBS-friendly recipes quickly and easily.

Chapter **17**

Setting Yourself Up for Low-FODMAP Success

I f you're living with irritable bowel syndrome (IBS) and you've decided to make a big dietary shift toward a low-FODMAP diet (or another dietary option outlined in Chapter 8), you may not be able to wake up one day and say "I'm going to switch my diet" and successfully implement it without any problems. Many people start out strong on the low-FODMAP diet, fully intending to stick with it, but then have difficulty maintaining the diet while managing a busy life. Plus, diet fatigue can occur when decisions about what to eat take a lot of effort, making you feel like giving up. You'll be much more successful if you reduce the burden on yourself by putting into place some plans and supports that allow you to give the diet a fair shot. With that said, the low-FODMAP diet can have rapid and dramatic effects on symptoms for some people, which is a powerful motivator in itself to stick to the diet for the required six to eight weeks.

TECHNICAL STUFF

FODMAP stands for *fermentable oligosaccharides, disaccharides, monosaccharides and polyols*. Read more about a low-FODMAP diet in Chapter 8.

Professional support from a registered dietitian is extremely valuable when embarking on a new diet (see the sidebar "How a registered dietitian can help with a low-FODMAP diet"). With or without a registered dietitian, however, you can take some simple actions to set yourself up for a dietary change and give yourself the best chance of success.

This chapter explains how to set up your environment to put you in the best position for a good outcome when you undertake a big dietary shift. You'll find practical advice to help you succeed, including shopping lists, ingredients to watch for, and a sample meal plan.

The advice in this chapter focuses on low–FODMAP, but it can also be adapted for other kinds of therapeutic diets for IBS.

TIP

Preparing to Change Your Diet

Before jumping in with the low–FODMAP diet, decide how long you plan to adhere to it — usually a minimum of four weeks and a maximum of 8 weeks. Look at your calendar and find a time period that spans the desired number of weeks when your routine is fairly normal, with no major travel or special events such as holidays. Mark the beginning of that time as the start date of the diet. Before that date arrives, here are some things that will help you prepare for success:

>> **Go to a pro.** If possible, attend an appointment in advance with a registered dietitian, who can give you meal suggestions and advice for your personal

situation and can answer questions along the way. (See the sidebar "How a registered dietitian can help with a low-FODMAP diet.")

>> **Inform important people in your life.** Tell your close family members and friends that you'll be starting a special medically recommended diet to improve your gut symptoms, and let them know any specific ways they can support you. The aim is not to change the way they eat, but to help keep you accountable for your own dietary change.

>> **Prepare a diet diary.** Obtain a new notebook, or print out copies of the chart you want to use as a diet diary and place the pages on a clipboard. Put the diary in an accessible location where you'll be reminded to fill it out every day with everything you eat and drink, along with approximate quantities. If you prefer, download a diet diary app (see Chapter 13).

>> **Budget for extra costs if necessary.** Gluten-free and other specialty foods, including specific fruits and vegetables that may be out of season, can increase your grocery costs. Budgeting for increased costs for the duration of your diet trial may be prudent; however, a registered dietitian may be able to provide tips on keeping your diet within budget.

>> **Download the Monash University FODMAP Diet app (see Chapter 13).** The Monash University FODMAP Diet app is the gold-standard tool for the low-FODMAP diet, allowing you look up the FODMAP content of many foods. (The app may not have all the foods you'd like to eat, but it has a wide variety that have been officially tested by experts at Monash University.)

TIP

Here are some ways you can shape your environment to increase your chances for success:

>> **Edit your fridge and cupboards.** Go through your refrigerator and cupboards to identify which items are okay for the low-FODMAP diet. If you live alone, you may want to toss out or hide items that are higher in FODMAPs. (If they're unopened, you may consider donating them to a local food bank.) However, if you live with other people who are continuing to consume the higher-FODMAP items, you may find it helpful to use a sticky dot or a piece of masking tape to mark the items you can safely consume. By marking these items, you may reduce the mental burden of figuring out what you can use every time you open the fridge or cupboard. (See the nearby sidebar for lists of common items that are and are not appropriate.)

>> **List what you can eat.** Make a list of snacks and simple meals that are allowed on the low-FODMAP diet, and that you enjoy, and post it in a visible place such as on the refrigerator.

>> **Consider making batches of commonly used sauces.** Look online for low-FODMAP versions of the sauces you commonly use, such as spaghetti

sauce and BBQ sauce. Consider making a large batch of sauce that you can freeze in smaller portions for easy use. (For example, freeze the sauce in an ice cube tray and transfer the frozen cubes to a freezer-safe container.)

» **Order specialty items.** Consider making an online order for some of the low-FODMAP specialty items you plan to use in your cooking: for example, garlic substitute or FODMAP-friendly prepared products. These items can be tricky to find at normal grocery stores, so you may be better off ordering them online before you start the diet.

COMMON FRIDGE AND PANTRY ITEMS THAT DO — AND DON'T — WORK ON A LOW-FODMAP DIET

Here are some common fridge and pantry items that aren't appropriate on a low-FODMAP diet:

Honey	Pasta sauce made with garlic or onion
Hummus	Relish
Jam (commercially made)	Salad dressings made with garlic or onion
Ketchup	Stock and stock cubes

And here are some common fridge and pantry items that you *can* eat on a low-FODMAP diet:

Apple cider vinegar	Red wine vinegar
Butter and margarine	Rice vinegar
Fish sauce	Sesame oil
Mayonnaise	Soy sauce (maximum 2 tablespoons)
Mustard	Vegetable oil
Nutritional yeast flakes	Worcestershire sauce
Olive oil	

Getting to Know Low-FODMAP Foods

Before you start low-FODMAP meal planning and grocery shopping, take some time to get your head around the list of lower- and higher-FODMAP foods.

REMEMBER

The low-FODMAP diet involves restricting certain types of carbohydrates. The major sources of these carbohydrates in a typical Western diet are wheat, milk, apples, pears, and stone fruits, and some other foods such as legumes, cauliflower, garlic, and onions. You can find a more detailed list of common high- and low-FODMAP foods in Chapter 8.

To properly implement a low-FODMAP diet, you'll need to get used to reading the ingredients lists on food packaging. In addition to avoiding the specific foods and ingredients you know will trigger your symptoms, you'll want to watch out for some of the higher-FODMAP ingredients on ingredient lists:

>> Chicory root

>> Fructo-oligosaccharides

>> Fructose or fructose syrup

>> Fruit juice concentrate

>> High-fructose corn syrup

>> Inulin

>> Isomalt

>> Lactose

>> Mannitol

>> Sorbitol

>> Xylitol

TIP

You may find yourself gravitating toward items with simpler ingredient lists, to reduce the burden of understanding what you're eating.

Ready-made low-FODMAP foods are also great options for simplifying your cooking. Several companies make low-FODMAP versions of prepared foods. These products tend to be available online and in some specialty health-food stores, and may be available in large grocery stores. The ready-made foods may include:

» Garlic-infused olive oil

» Granola bars

» Ketchup

» Marinades

» Pasta sauce

» Salad dressings

» Salsa

TIP

Companies that don't specialize in low-FODMAP foods may also have individual products that are certified as low-FODMAP. Look for the green FODMAP Friendly logo on the label (see Figure 17-1). All the FODMAP Friendly certified products and many tested ingredients are also searchable through the FODMAP Friendly app (go to https://fodmapfriendly.com/app). Remember that a food item may contain some FODMAPs and still qualify for the low-FODMAP certification if the amount is low enough.

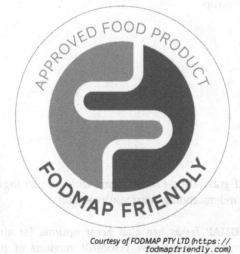

FIGURE 17-1:
Look for the FODMAP Friendly logo to find food products certified as low-FODMAP.

Courtesy of FODMAP PTY LTD (https://fodmapfriendly.com)

Another option, depending on where you live, may be delivery meal kits or frozen meals that are specifically created to be low-FODMAP.

Planning Low-FODMAP Meals

Before you start on a low-FODMAP diet, planning out at least one week of meals can help you get a feel for which foods are allowed and not allowed on the diet. Mapping out what you'll eat can save you a lot of time and prevent panic when you're behind schedule and ravenously hungry. Table 17-1 shows an example one-week meal plan, which uses some of the low-FODMAP recipes in Chapters 18 through 21.

TIP

Be realistic when you create your meal plan, and base it on your normal eating habits. For example, if you tend to eat cereal with fruit for breakfast, then you can plan to continue eating cereal with fruit — albeit a low-FODMAP cereal, with low-FODMAP fruit. If you usually cook homemade dinners, then plan to continue cooking low-FODMAP dinners. But if you tend to eat convenient foods that don't require cooking, base your meal plan around low-FODMAP versions of those foods instead.

REMEMBER

You don't need to reinvent the wheel — or the meal plan. If you normally have a weekly pasta night, you can swap out the wheat pasta with gluten-free pasta and low-FODMAP sauce. Start with what you normally do and adapt as needed.

In addition to the recipes in this book, you may be able to find great recipes from the many low-FODMAP recipe blogs. If you're using the recipes from these blogs, however, take a moment to scan the ingredients list and double-check the FODMAP content using the Monash University FODMAP Diet app (see Chapter 13), because some bloggers have been known to make mistakes on the FODMAP content of the ingredients.

Good recipe blogs include the following (but still double-check the ingredients):

>> **A Little Bit Yummy:** https://alittlebityummy.com/recipes

>> **FODMAP Everyday:** www.fodmapeveryday.com/recipes

>> **For A Digestive Peace of Mind:** http://blog.katescarlata.com

>> **Monash University Low FODMAP Recipes:** www.monashfodmap.com/recipe

>> **Vanessa Hummel:** www.vanessahummel.com/blog/categories/recipe

TABLE 17-1 Sample Low-FODMAP Five-Day Meal Plan

	Monday	Tuesday	Wednesday	Thursday	Friday
Breakfast	½ cup cooked oatmeal with 1 teaspoon maple syrup and 1 teaspoon cinnamon ½ cup blueberries blended into a smoothie with 1 cup lactose-free milk or almond milk	1-egg omelet with ½ cup spinach and 1 ounce cheddar cheese 1 slice sourdough bread 1 clementine orange	Yogurt parfait made with ½ cup lactose-free yogurt; 10 almonds, crushed; and 4 or 5 fresh strawberries, sliced	2 Pumpkin Spice Oatmeal Muffins (Chapter 21) 1 banana	Strawberry smoothie bowl made by blending 1 cup strawberries, frozen; ½ banana, frozen; 1 cup spinach; 1 tablespoon chia seeds; and ½ cup almond milk (plus water if needed for thinning)
Snack	1 or 2 hard-boiled eggs 2 kiwis	2 rice cakes with 2 tablespoons natural peanut or almond butter	½ cup wheat pretzels 1 tablespoon natural peanut butter	10 rice crackers with 1 ounce of lactose-free cheese (for example, old cheddar or Gouda)	2 Chocolate Chip Chia Energy Balls (Chapter 21)
Lunch	Low-FODMAP veggie pasta salad made by combining 1 cup cooked gluten-free pasta with 3 cherry tomatoes, ¼ cup chopped cucumber, 5 black olives, and 1 tablespoon chopped fresh basil, topped with a low-FODMAP dressing	Grilled chicken salad made with 3 to 4 ounces of grilled chicken breast, up to 1.5 cups mixed greens (lettuce, spinach, and/or arugula), ¼ cup chopped cucumber, 3 tablespoons grated carrot, and 3 medium cherry tomatoes, topped with a low-FODMAP dressing	Tuna salad lettuce wraps made with 3 ounces canned tuna, 1 tablespoon mayonnaise, and 1 cup lettuce on a gluten-free wrap	Nicoise salad made with 1 boiled egg, 2.5 ounces (71 grams) steamed green beans, 3 cherry tomatoes, ¼ cup black olives, and 3 ounces canned tuna, topped with a low-FODMAP vinaigrette dressing	Mediterranean quinoa bowl made by combining 1 cup cooked quinoa, 1 grilled chicken breast, ¼ cup chopped cucumber, 3 cherry tomatoes, 5 black olives, 1 cup baby spinach, 1 tablespoon chopped fresh parsley, 2 tablespoons olive oil, and a squeeze of lemon

	Monday	Tuesday	Wednesday	Thursday	Friday
Snack	¼ cup chopped bell pepper ¼ cup walnuts (about 10 halves)	1 square dark chocolate ½ cup fresh blueberries	½ cup chopped cucumber Low-FODMAP ranch dip, made by combining 1 cup lactose-free yogurt, ¼ tablespoon fresh dill, and 1 teaspoon lemon juice	¾ cup cantaloupe ¼ cup pecans (about 10 halves)	1 mozzarella cheese stick 1 mandarin orange
Dinner	Lemony Kale Chicken (Chapter 19) 1 cup white rice	Miso Soba Noodles with Salmon (Chapter 19) 1 cup steamed green beans	Gluten-free pasta with commercial low-FODMAP tomato sauce Up to 1½ cups mixed-greens salad	Chicken and Feta Patties (Chapter 19) 6 roasted baby potatoes Up to 1½ cups mixed-greens salad	Pork and Cabbage Rice-Paper Wraps (Chapter 19) Up to 1½ cups mixed-greens salad
Snack	Popcorn	Tortilla chips with commercial low-FODMAP salsa	½ ounce dark chocolate 10 almonds	Strawberry Chia Pudding (Chapter 19)	Rice puff cereal with lactose-free milk and ⅓ banana

Grocery Shopping for Success

Armed with a menu plan for your low–FODMAP diet, and with the start date approaching, it's time to shop for all the items you need to implement your plan.

TIP

Here are some tips to make your low–FODMAP grocery shopping go smoothly:

>> **Choose a grocery store that has a good variety of items.** Wholesale stores such as Costco that stock inconsistent inventory aren't the best places to look when you have a list of more specific items for your diet plan. Instead, shop somewhere with a range of items, including specialty items, so you'll be able to find what you need.

>> **Allow yourself extra time.** The first few times you shop for a low-FODMAP diet, plan to shop at off-peak times and allow yourself extra time to browse and compare options.

>> **Avoid buying large quantities of a product when you first start a low-FODMAP diet.** Finding foods that work for you can take some trial and error. If you don't typically consume the product, choose a smaller package or jar at first so you've spent less money and there's less waste if you decide to switch to something else.

>> **Focus on fresh, whole produce when you shop.** Stock up on fresh produce that's low-FODMAP and easy to prepare. Vegetables such as bell peppers, carrots, cucumbers, green beans, lettuce, spinach, and zucchini are great to have on hand. Fruits such as bananas, blueberries, cantaloupe, grapes, honeydew melon, kiwifruits, oranges, and strawberries are good choices, too.

>> **Don't be afraid to buy frozen.** Frozen low-FODMAP vegetables and fruits can be convenient when fresh produce isn't available or isn't within your budget. These frozen items pack a good nutritional punch and may help avoid waste.

Cooking Low-FODMAP Meals

When the start date of your low-FODMAP diet arrives, it's time to dig in and implement your meal plan. Your first week on the diet may be a time of delicious, tummy-friendly eating if you successfully stick to the diet.

TIP

Here are some tips to make your low-FODMAP cooking more successful:

>> **Adhere to the recipe.** Even if you're a cook who likes to improvise from time to time, stick to the recipes at first. By following the recipes exactly, you'll be able to get a sense of the ingredients and amounts that will allow you to stay below the target low-FODMAP threshold.

>> **Be generous with your use of low-FODMAP seasonings.** You can add delicious flavor to dishes with many herbs and spices, without needing to fall back on the old standby, garlic. Basil, black pepper, cilantro, ginger, oregano, paprika, rosemary, sage, thyme, and turmeric are all low-FODMAP options that you can use in your recipes. Asafetida, commonly used in Indian cuisine, adds a subtle onion and garlic flavor without FODMAPs.

>> **Incorporate low-FODMAP onion and garlic flavors.** Shallot- or garlic-infused olive oil adds flavor to dressings. The green parts of leeks or green onions are safe to consume on a low-FODMAP diet, and provide a subtle onion flavor.

>> **Stock up on stock.** Real stock adds richness and flavor to so many recipes, from soups and stews to risotto and sauces. Make your own chicken or vegetable stock and freeze it in recipe-size portions so you have it on hand.

>> **Make a batch.** Prepare a larger batch of some meals so that you can either use the leftovers that week or freeze some for an easy meal later on.

>> **Use time-saving tools.** Prepare meals using kitchen tools such as a rice cooker, a slow cooker, or an Instant Pot to save time.

Monitoring Your Progress

If you've done all the preparations and started on the low-FODMAP diet, congratulations! You're embarking on the most scientifically backed treatment for getting IBS symptoms under control. (That's not to say it's the one and only treatment you're likely to need, though — see Chapters 9 through 12 for other effective IBS interventions.)

You may notice a difference in your symptoms right away, or you may not. To ensure you get the most out of your efforts, keep a record of what you're eating every day, and also keep track of your symptoms. If you successfully reduce your symptoms, your diet diary will provide a list of foods that are fine for you to continue eating as you work to expand your diet beyond low-FODMAP. And if you're not successful, then you have the option to enlist a professional to go through your food diary and perhaps help you figure out what foods or food components may be triggering your symptoms. If you continue to adjust the diet based on your diet diary and it still isn't working for you, dietary change may not be the ideal treatment option for you — but you'll have the records to prove it.

Chapter **18**

Soups and Salads

With or without irritable bowel syndrome (IBS), you help support your gut health when you eat a diverse array of foods — especially plant foods. Soups and salads make some of the best kinds of meals because they tend to be easy ways to incorporate a wide range of healthy ingredients into a single dish.

In addition, many soups and salads are very versatile, making them ideal for tailoring to specific dietary needs. All the soups and salads in this chapter are low-FODMAP, but if you identify an ingredient that's a trigger for you, you can usually leave it out or swap it for a similar ingredient that you tolerate better. And if you have an extra ingredient in your fridge that you know you tolerate and that fits with the recipe, you can feel free to add it. A handful of pumpkin seeds, some shredded fennel, a pinch of chia seeds — customize as you see fit!

TECHNICAL STUFF

FODMAP stands for *fermentable oligosaccharides, disaccharides, monosaccharides and polyols*. Read more about a low-FODMAP diet in Chapter 8.

In this chapter, we provide recipes for some nourishing low-FODMAP soups, followed by a selection of salads that are IBS-friendly and can serve as a main meal that incorporates diverse ingredients.

Concocting Soups That Nourish the Gut

Soups are excellent comfort food. Especially during cold weather, nothing beats the coziness of a pot of soup simmering on the stove — not to mention the nourishment you get from enjoying the soup itself. Normally, many soups rely on garlic or onion (which are not low-FODMAP) as base flavors, but the recipes in this chapter show that you can definitely make delicious soups without these ingredients.

The following recipes are found in this section:

>> **Creamy Kabocha Soup:** This soup is mellow and creamy, and it tastes even better when reheated. Portion it out in jars and store in the fridge for an easy lunch to take to work.

>> **Lentil Carrot Soup:** This soup is both bright and hearty, with richness added through miso and tomato paste.

>> **Corn and Millet Soup:** This mild soup has the comforting flavor of toasted millet and is easy on the belly.

THE LOW-FODMAP BROTH PROBLEM

Broth is an essential ingredient of soup. Normally when making a soup, you either buy a commercial broth product (a carton or can of broth or bouillon) or make a homemade broth infused with garlic and onion. The problem is that on a low-FODMAP diet, garlic and onion have to be avoided, so almost none of the commercial broths or broth recipes are suitable. So, how can you make delicious, rich soups with this broth constraint?

With a little creativity, you can make delicious soups even without garlic and onion. Try these ideas for increasing richness and flavor when water is called for in this chapter's soup recipes:

- When you boil potatoes, reserve the water you drain off the potatoes and use it as a broth. This adds depth and mouthfeel to the soup.

- After shaving the kernels off a cob of corn, boil the cobs for 10 to 15 minutes and reserve the water as a savory broth.

- Miso paste (used in several recipes in this chapter) added to water makes a rich, savory broth.

- Create your own bone broth. (See this chapter's sidebar "DIY bone broth.")

Lentil Carrot Soup

PREP TIME: 10 MIN	COOK TIME: 1 HR 10 MIN	YIELD: 4 SERVINGS

INGREDIENTS

5 medium carrots, peeled

2 tablespoons (15 mL) extra-virgin olive oil (garlic-infused, if desired), divided

Pinch of white sugar

1 tablespoon (15 mL) green onion tops, finely chopped

2 tablespoons (30 mL) celery, finely chopped

6 cups (1.5 L) water

1½ teaspoons (7.5 mL) salt

Pinch of black pepper

2 teaspoons (10 mL) dried oregano

½ teaspoon (2.5 mL) dried sage

1 tablespoon (15 mL) miso

2 tablespoons (30 mL) tomato paste

1 tablespoon (15 mL) nutritional yeast

¾ cup (180 mL) canned lentils, drained and rinsed

2 cups (500 mL) curly green kale, destemmed and chopped

1 tablespoon (15 mL) lemon juice

Fresh parsley, chopped, for garnish (optional)

DIRECTIONS

1 Preheat the oven to 425°F (220°C).

2 Line a baking sheet with parchment. Place the whole carrots onto the prepared sheet and drizzle with 1 tablespoon of the olive oil. Sprinkle a pinch of sugar over the top. Bake for 40 minutes or until the carrots are slightly browned. (They may be unevenly cooked, which is fine because they'll continue to cook in the broth.) Set aside to cool.

3 In a large pot over medium-high heat, add the remaining 1 tablespoon of olive oil along with the green onion tops and celery. Cook for around 2 minutes, until the celery is softened.

4 To the pot, add the water, salt, pepper, oregano, sage, miso, tomato paste, and nutritional yeast. Stir briefly; then add the lentils and kale. Chop the roasted carrots and add them to the pot.

5 Bring to a boil, then reduce the heat to medium-low and simmer for a few more minutes, until the kale has softened to your desired texture. Remove from the heat.

6 Add the lemon juice and stir. Serve the soup into bowls and garnish with fresh parsley if desired.

PER SERVING: *Calories 177 (From Fat 69); Fat 8g (Saturated 1g); Cholesterol 0mg; Sodium 1025mg; Carbohydrate 23g (Dietary Fiber 7g); Protein 7g.*

TIP: Red miso works best for this recipe. Adjust the amount of miso to taste, based on the saltiness of the variety you're using.

NOTE: Lentils are considered low-FODMAP at a serving of less than ½ cup (cooked or canned).

DIY BONE BROTH

Real bone broth makes an excellent base for soups, or even to sip on its own when your symptoms are flaring up. Because most commercially available broths contain garlic or onion, you may not be able to use them when following a low-FODMAP diet. A great option is to make your own bone broth, leaving out the garlic and onion.

The basic technique for making chicken broth is to put the bones, skin, and gristle from a cooked chicken into a large pot and cover with cold water. Throw in some celery leaves, green leek tops, chopped fennel bulb, or carrot peelings for flavor if desired. You can also add a sachet of spices such as peppercorns, sprigs of thyme, or a bay leaf. Bring to a rolling boil; then reduce the heat to low. Skim any foam off the top. Cover and simmer on low for 5 hours or more. Remove the pot from the heat, and when slightly cooled, strain out all the solids. Chill the broth in the refrigerator overnight; then skim the fat off the top and discard it. Either keep the broth in the fridge for up to five days to use as needed, or divide it into freezer-safe containers (leaving room for expansion) and freeze. If you prefer to make a broth from beef bones, replace the chicken parts with around 5 pounds of beef bones (including marrow bones or bones with some meat attached), and roast them at 425°F (220°C) for about half an hour before proceeding with the broth recipe.

Creamy Kabocha Soup

PREP TIME: 5 MIN	COOK TIME: 1 HR 10 MIN	YIELD: 4 SERVINGS

INGREDIENTS

1 medium kabocha squash (around 2½ pounds), whole

1 cup (250 mL) canned regular-fat coconut milk

2 cups (500 mL) water

1½ teaspoons (7.5 mL) salt

Pinch of black pepper

1 tablespoon (15 mL) curry powder

½ teaspoon (2.5 mL) ground nutmeg

1 teaspoon (5 mL) Dijon mustard

DIRECTIONS

1 Preheat the oven to 350°F (180°C).

2 Line a baking sheet with parchment. Cut the squash in half and place it face-down on the prepared sheet. Bake for 45 minutes or until the skin can be easily pierced with a fork. Remove from the oven and cool.

3 Turn the squash halves over and lightly scrape out the seeds and pulp, discarding them. Using a spoon, scrape the orange flesh of the squash out of the peel and mash lightly with a fork.

4 In a large pot over medium-high heat, combine 3 cups of the squash with the coconut milk, water, salt, pepper, curry powder, nutmeg, and mustard.

5 Bring to a boil, and then reduce the heat to medium-low and simmer for 5 minutes.

6 Remove from the heat and allow the soup to cool slightly. Using an immersion blender, blend the soup until it has a smooth, creamy texture.

PER SERVING: *Calories 231 (From Fat 113); Fat 13g (Saturated 11g); Cholesterol 0mg; Sodium 903mg; Carbohydrate 32g (Dietary Fiber 5g); Protein 4g.*

Corn and Millet Soup

PREP TIME: 5 MIN	COOK TIME: 45 MIN	YIELD: 4 SERVINGS

INGREDIENTS

⅔ cup (160 mL) uncooked millet, rinsed

2 strips uncooked bacon, chopped

1 tablespoon (15 mL) extra-virgin olive oil

¼ cup (60 mL) celery, finely chopped

6 cups (1.5 L) water

2 teaspoons (10 mL) salt

Pinch of black pepper

1 teaspoon (5 mL) dried thyme

½ teaspoon (2.5 mL) dried sage

Two 7-ounce (200 mL) cans corn niblets, drained

1 tablespoon (15 mL) miso

DIRECTIONS

1 In a small frying pan over medium-high heat, toast the millet for 2 to 3 minutes, stirring constantly, until aromatic. Remove from the heat and set aside.

2 In a large pot over medium-high heat, fry the bacon for about 5minutes until slightly browned. Add the olive oil and celery and continue frying for another minute, until the celery is slightly softened.

3 Add the water, salt, pepper, thyme, sage, and corn. Add the millet and stir.

4 Bring to a boil and continue to boil for 5 minutes. Reduce the heat to medium-low, add the miso, and then cover the pot.

5 Simmer for around 15 more minutes, until the millet is fully cooked and soft.

6 Divide into bowls and serve.

PER SERVING: *Calories 270 (From Fat 95); Fat 11g (Saturated 3g); Cholesterol 8mg; Sodium 1427mg; Carbohydrate 39g (Dietary Fiber 4g); Protein 7g.*

Making IBS-Friendly Salads

Typically a salad is something that people with IBS avoid because many common salad ingredients, such as lettuce and raw tomato, can cause gut symptoms, especially if eaten in high amounts. But if you have a broad definition of *salad*, you'll find that many salads can be made IBS-friendly. This section is filled with salads that are so hearty and delicious, they can serve as an entire meal. Each salad, in stark contrast with the stereotypical side salad of wilted iceberg lettuce and mealy tomato, incorporates a variety of fresh and nourishing ingredients to help you increase the diversity of foods in your diet.

The salads in this chapter are:

>> **Vermicelli Chicken Salad:** This hearty salad has bold flavor and makes a great meal in the summertime.

>> **Soba Salad with Peanut-Lime Dressing:** Better than takeout, this salad tastes rich and delicious with its creamy peanut and lime dressing.

>> **Moroccan Roasted Vegetable Salad:** This nourishing salad, made with loads of roasted vegetables, makes a comforting meal with its mixture of warm spices.

>> **Halloumi and Arugula Salad:** This salad, topped with golden-brown fried halloumi cheese, makes a quick and satisfying meal.

>> **Potato Bacon Salad:** The tanginess of the dressing and fresh parsley offsets the mellow flavors of potatoes and bacon, perfectly balancing the flavors in this salad.

Potato Bacon Salad

INGREDIENTS

3 cups (750 mL) uncooked potatoes, chopped into bite-size pieces with skin on

3 slices uncooked thick-cut bacon, chopped

3 tablespoons (45 mL) apple cider vinegar

1 tablespoon (15 mL) yellow mustard

1 teaspoon (5 mL) salt

Pinch of black pepper

1 tablespoon (15 mL) white sugar

2 teaspoons (10 mL) extra-virgin olive oil

¼ cup (60 mL) fresh parsley, finely chopped

1 tablespoon (15 mL) green onion tops, finely chopped

DIRECTIONS

1 Place the potatoes in a medium pot and cover with cold water. Heat on medium-high and bring to a boil. Continue to boil for 3 to 4 minutes, or until the potatoes are fork-tender. Remove from the heat and drain. Transfer to a large bowl.

2 In a medium skillet over medium-high heat, cook the bacon for 8 to 10 minutes, or until desired crispness is reached. Transfer the bacon pieces to a plate lined with a paper towel.

3 In a medium bowl, combine the apple cider vinegar, mustard, salt, pepper, sugar, and olive oil. Mix well.

4 Pour the dressing over the potatoes. Add the parsley and green onion tops and toss. Serve warm or chilled.

PER SERVING: *Calories 270 (From Fat 139); Fat 15g (Saturated 5g); Cholesterol 19mg; Sodium 878mg; Carbohydrate 26g (Dietary Fiber 2g); Protein 6g.*

TIP: New potatoes are the best ones to use for this recipe because they have a firm, waxy texture that works well in a potato salad. You can also save the water used to boil the potatoes to use as a soup broth.

Vermicelli Chicken Salad

PREP TIME: 5 MIN	COOK TIME: 15 MIN	YIELD: 4 SERVINGS

INGREDIENTS

1 teaspoon (5 mL) plus
2 tablespoons (30 mL)
extra-virgin olive oil, divided

1 teaspoon (5 mL) salt, divided

1 pound (450 g) uncooked
chicken breasts, chopped into
1-inch cubes

5 oz (150 g) uncooked rice
vermicelli noodles

3 leaves Romaine
lettuce, chopped

1 medium carrot, peeled
and shredded

1 tablespoon (15 mL) cilantro,
finely chopped

3 tablespoons (45 mL) apple
cider vinegar

2 tablespoons (30 mL)
sesame oil

Pinch of black pepper

2 tablespoons (30 mL) sugar

Sesame seeds for garnish
(optional)

DIRECTIONS

1 In a large skillet over medium-high heat, add 1 teaspoon of the olive oil, ½ teaspoon of the salt, and the chicken breasts. Cook for 8 to 10 minutes, until the chicken breasts are fully cooked and slightly browned. Remove from the heat, drain any remaining juices, and set aside.

2 Place the vermicelli noodles in a large bowl and cover with boiling water. Let them sit for around 3 minutes, or until tender. Drain, rinse with cold water, and transfer to a large bowl.

3 To the bowl, add the lettuce, carrot, cilantro, and cooked chicken; toss gently.

4 In a medium bowl, combine the apple cider vinegar, the remaining 2 tablespoons of olive oil, the sesame oil, the remaining ½ teaspoon of salt, the pepper, and the sugar. Mix well.

5 Pour the dressing over the ingredients in the large bowl and mix. Garnish with sesame seeds if desired and serve.

PER SERVING: *Calories 425 (From Fat 161); Fat 18g (Saturated 3g); Cholesterol 73mg; Sodium 791mg; Carbohydrate 38g (Dietary Fiber 1g); Protein 26g.*

Soba Salad with Peanut-Lime Dressing

PREP TIME: 10 MIN	COOK TIME: 5 MIN	YIELD: 4 SERVINGS

INGREDIENTS

¼ cup (60 mL) salted natural peanut butter, smooth

1 tablespoon (15 mL) tamari (gluten-free)

1 teaspoon (5 mL) maple syrup

1 teaspoon (5 mL) ginger, minced

1 teaspoon (5 mL) sesame oil

2 tablespoons (30 mL) lime juice

1 tablespoon (15 mL) warm water

7 ounces (200 g) 100 percent buckwheat soba

1 cup (250 mL) red cabbage, shredded

1 cup (250 mL) carrot, peeled and shredded

½ cup (125 mL) cucumber, diced

2 tablespoons (30 mL) cilantro, finely chopped

Peanuts for garnish, optional

DIRECTIONS

1 In a medium bowl, combine the peanut butter, soy sauce, maple syrup, ginger, sesame oil, and lime juice. Mix gently. Add the warm water and mix until the dressing is a smooth consistency.

2 Fill a medium pot with water and bring to a boil. Add the soba and cook for around 4 minutes, or until the noodles are tender. Drain and rinse in cold water; then transfer to a large bowl.

3 Immediately pour the dressing over the noodles and mix to prevent sticking.

4 Add the cabbage, carrot, cucumber, and cilantro. Toss to combine.

5 Garnish with peanuts if desired. Serve warm or chilled.

PER SERVING: *Calories 300 (From Fat 88); Fat 10g (Saturated 2g); Cholesterol 0mg; Sodium 745mg; Carbohydrate 47g (Dietary Fiber 2g); Protein 12g.*

NOTE: When buying soba, check the package to make sure they're made with 100 percent buckwheat flour. Some varieties contain added wheat flour, which is not low-FODMAP. If 100 percent buckwheat soba are not available, you can use vermicelli noodles instead.

Moroccan Roasted Vegetable Salad

PREP TIME: 15 MIN	COOK TIME: 30 MIN	YIELD: 4 SERVINGS

INGREDIENTS

1 cup (250 mL) zucchini, chopped

1½ cups (375 mL) uncooked butternut squash, peeled and chopped

1 cup (250 mL) carrot, peeled and chopped

3 tablespoons (45 mL) extra-virgin olive oil, divided

2 pinches of black pepper, divided

1 cup (250 mL) water

½ cup (125 mL) uncooked quinoa

1 teaspoon (5 mL) cinnamon

1 teaspoon (5 mL) cumin

½ teaspoon (2.5 mL) ground nutmeg

1½ teaspoons (7.5 mL) ground ginger

½ teaspoon (2.5 mL) smoked paprika

½ teaspoon (2.5 mL) salt

1 teaspoon (5 mL) lemon zest

2 tablespoons (30 mL) lemon juice

2 cups (500 mL) baby spinach leaves

½ cup (125 mL) canned chickpeas, drained and rinsed

DIRECTIONS

1 Preheat the oven to 400°F (200°C).

2 Line a baking sheet with parchment. Place the zucchini, squash, and carrot on the prepared sheet and drizzle with 1 tablespoon of the olive oil and 1 pinch of the black pepper. Bake for 15 minutes; then remove from the oven and toss. Bake for an additional 15 minutes, until the vegetables are browned and fork-tender.

3 While the vegetables are roasting, combine the water and quinoa in a medium pot over medium-high heat. Bring to a boil; then reduce the heat to medium and simmer for around 13 minutes, stirring occasionally, until most of the water is absorbed. Remove from the heat; then cover and let the quinoa sit for 10 minutes.

4 In a small bowl, combine the cinnamon, cumin, nutmeg, ginger, paprika, salt, and the remaining 1 pinch of black pepper. Mix to combine.

5 To the spices, add the lemon zest, lemon juice, and the remaining 2 tablespoons of olive oil. Mix well.

6 In a large bowl, combine the roasted vegetables, the cooked quinoa, the baby spinach, and the chickpeas. Pour the dressing over the top and toss to combine. Serve warm or chilled.

PER SERVING: *Calories 264 (From Fat 113); Fat 13g (Saturated 2g); Cholesterol 0mg; Sodium 406mg; Carbohydrate 33g (Dietary Fiber 6g); Protein 7g.*

NOTE: Although chickpeas contain galacto-oligosaccharides, which are generally not recommended on a low-FODMAP diet, a small serving of around ¼ cup of chickpeas per meal is considered low-FODMAP. The amount in this recipe, spread over 4 servings, is under the low-FODMAP threshold.

Halloumi and Arugula Salad

INGREDIENTS

4 cups (1 L) arugula leaves

1 cup (250 mL) cherry tomatoes, chopped

¼ cup (60 mL) kalamata olives, pitted and chopped

½ cup (125 mL) canned chickpeas, drained

½ cup (125 mL) red pepper, chopped

¼ cup (60 mL) plus 1 teaspoon (5 mL) extra-virgin olive oil

2 tablespoons (30 mL) balsamic vinegar

½ teaspoon (2.5 mL) dried oregano

1 tablespoon (30 mL) Dijon mustard

¼ teaspoon (1 mL) salt

Pinch of black pepper

2 tablespoons (30 mL) plain coconut-based yogurt

1 tablespoon (15 mL) maple syrup

One 9-ounce (250 g) package halloumi, cubed

DIRECTIONS

1 In a large bowl, combine the arugula, cherry tomatoes, olives, chickpeas, and red pepper.

2 In a small bowl, combine ¼ cup of the olive oil, the balsamic vinegar, the oregano, the mustard, the salt, the pepper, the yogurt, and the maple syrup. Mix well.

3 In a medium skillet over medium-high heat, add the remaining 1 teaspoon of olive oil along with the halloumi. Cook for 3 to 4 minutes, stirring occasionally, until the halloumi is browned.

4 Transfer the halloumi to the large bowl. Pour the dressing over the top and toss to combine. Serve immediately.

PER SERVING: *Calories 426 (From Fat 296); Fat 33g (Saturated 14g); Cholesterol 45mg; Sodium 1032mg; Carbohydrate 17g (Dietary Fiber 4g); Protein 18g.*

TIP: If you don't plan to eat the whole salad right away, omit the arugula from the large bowl of other ingredients. Add the desired amount of arugula to an individual serving bowl and add the rest of the salad on top. This ensures that the arugula remains fresher until you consume it.

Chapter **19**

Main Dishes

I f you're on the low-FODMAP diet, you may be avoiding certain types of carbohydrates, but luckily, you have many choices for high-protein foods that can create hearty, satisfying meals.

Typically, a cook would kick-start the flavor of a main dish with some garlic or onion frying in a pan, but those foods are not low-FODMAP. Fortunately, many flavorful ingredients can be used to create tasty dishes in the absence of these staples.

TECHNICAL STUFF

FODMAP stands for *fermentable oligosaccharides, disaccharides, monosaccharides and polyols.* Read more about a low-FODMAP diet in Chapter 8.

This chapter features recipes for main dishes that are low in FODMAP ingredients and, therefore, easy on your digestion. The first section offers lighter dishes based on fish, seafood, and tofu; the second section offers meat-based dishes.

Creating Main Dishes from Fish, Seafood, and Tofu

Fish and seafood are superstar foods in many healthy diet patterns such as the Mediterranean diet. They're a good source of high-quality protein and heart-healthy omega-3 fatty acids. Fresh fish and seafood is ideal, but frozen versions work perfectly well for these recipes — plus, they may be easier to come by (and sometimes easier on your pocketbook).

Tofu is another light-tasting protein to use in your main dishes. Moderate amounts of firm or extra-firm tofu are acceptable on a low-FODMAP diet, and you can often substitute tofu cubes for either the fish or the meat in this chapter's recipes.

The recipes in this section are as follows:

» **Tuna Sweet Potato Patties:** These hearty tuna patties have protein and slower-burning carbohydrates all in one serving. They taste great as leftovers, too.

» **Shrimp, Pepper, and Pineapple Skewers with Pesto Rice:** These showstopping skewers make a fresh and tasty meal alongside pesto rice.

» **Miso Soba Noodles with Salmon:** This tasty dish is the ultimate low-FODMAP comfort food to enjoy for lunch or dinner.

» **Ginger Tofu Noodle Bowls:** These light-tasting noodle bowls make a nice, easy meal when you're short on time.

» **Sweet-and-Sour Pineapple Fish:** A super easy and tasty sauce that complements your choice of fish.

GARLIC AND ONION FLAVORS WITHOUT THE TUMMY TROUBLE

Garlic is a flavorful food that's not permitted on the low-FODMAP diet (at least in the beginning stages) because of its high fructan content. But that doesn't mean you have to go without delicious garlic flavor. One alternative is a spice called asafetida (also known by the less appealing name "stinking gum"), which is a powdered resin from ferula, an herb. A pinch of this spice can approximate the pungent flavor of garlic. If available, you may also seek out a low-FODMAP garlic replacer product (made from maltodextrin with garlic flavoring, for example). You can find this kind of product at specialty food stores or order it online.

Another option is to use garlic-infused olive oil. You may be able to buy premade garlic-infused olive oil, but it's also easy to make your own: Place ¼ cup extra-virgin olive oil in a small saucepan over medium heat. Add 2 to 4 garlic cloves that have been peeled and cut in half. Bring to a simmer, and continue cooking gently for about 5 minutes, until the garlic oil becomes fragrant. Remove from the heat. Take out the garlic pieces from the oil and discard them. Use the oil anywhere you'd use olive oil. Store your garlic-infused olive oil in the fridge, and bring it to room temperature before using.

To add the flavor of onion to a dish, use green onion tops or scallions. The green parts are low in FODMAPs, but the bulb (the white part) is high-FODMAP and should be avoided when following a low-FODMAP diet. Chives and leeks (again, only the green tops) are other alternatives to help you add flavor to dishes. If a dish calls for caramelized onions, chopped fennel bulb can be used as a safe low-FODMAP alternative.

Tuna Sweet Potato Patties

PREP TIME: 10 MIN	COOK TIME: 12 MIN	YIELD: 4 SERVINGS (8 PATTIES)

INGREDIENTS

2 cups (500 mL) white or orange sweet potato, peeled and cut into 1-inch chunks (about 1½ medium potatoes)

Two 5-ounce (185 g) cans chunk light tuna, drained

3 eggs

½ teaspoon (2.5 mL) salt

Pinch of black pepper

⅓ cup (80 mL) red pepper, finely chopped

1 tablespoon (15 mL) green onion tops, finely chopped

1 tablespoon (15 mL) extra-virgin olive oil

¼ cup (60 mL) sour cream

¼ cup (60 mL) mayonnaise

1 tablespoon (15 mL) lemon juice

1 teaspoon (5 mL) sugar

1 teaspoon (5 mL) Dijon mustard

3 tablespoons (45 mL) chopped gherkins

DIRECTIONS

1 Fill a medium pot with water and bring to a boil over high heat.

2 Add the sweet potato, reduce the heat slightly, and boil for 5 to 7 minutes, until the potatoes are fork-tender. Drain and return the potatoes to the pot.

3 Roughly mash the potatoes using a potato masher.

4 To the slightly cooled potatoes, add the tuna, eggs, salt, black pepper, red pepper, and green onion tops. Mix well.

5 Heat the olive oil over medium-high heat in a large frying pan. Add the peppers and fry for approximately 1 minute until slightly softened.

6 Remove the peppers from the frying pan using a slotted spoon and add them to the potato mixture. Mix well.

7 For each patty, take about ⅓ cup of the mixture and place it in the frying pan, flattening gently. Add a dash more olive oil if needed for frying. Cook the patties for around 4 minutes on each side, until well browned.

8 In a small bowl, combine the sour cream, mayonnaise, lemon juice, sugar, mustard, and gherkins and mix. Serve the patties with this dipping sauce.

PER SERVING: *Calories 318 (From Fat 140); Fat 16g (Saturated 4g); Cholesterol 191mg; Sodium 752mg; Carbohydrate 20g (Dietary Fiber 2g); Protein 24g.*

NOTE: These patties go well on top of a green salad dressed with a light vinaigrette. To stay under the safe limit for FODMAP intake of sweet potato, be sure to consume no more than 3 patties in one sitting.

TIP: If you don't want to use the suggested dipping sauce, turn up the flavor of these patties with Asian-style sweet chili sauce, which is considered low-FODMAP at a serving of around 2 tablespoons.

Shrimp, Pepper, and Pineapple Skewers with Pesto Rice

PREP TIME: 15 MIN	COOK TIME: 20 MIN	YIELD: 4 SERVINGS (8 SKEWERS)

INGREDIENTS

1 cup (250 mL) fresh basil leaves, chopped

2 cups (500 mL) baby spinach leaves, chopped

½ cup (125 mL) pine nuts

¼ cup (60 mL) grated Parmesan cheese

¼ cup (60 mL) plus 1 tablespoon (15 mL) extra-virgin olive oil, divided

1 tablespoon (15 mL) plus 2 teaspoons (10 mL) lemon juice, divided

¾ teaspoon (3.5 mL) salt, divided

Pinch of black pepper

1 cup (250 mL) jasmine rice, uncooked

2 cups (500 mL) water

1 teaspoon (5 mL) balsamic vinegar

24 one-inch chunks fresh pineapple

24 one-inch pieces red pepper

24 raw jumbo shrimp, peeled (if frozen, thawed and drained)

DIRECTIONS

1 Preheat the oven to 350°F (180°C).

2 In a blender (or small bowl if using an immersion blender), combine the basil, spinach, pine nuts, Parmesan cheese, ¼ cup of the olive oil, 1 tablespoon of the lemon juice, ½ teaspoon of the salt, and the pepper. Blend until it creates a smooth pesto.

3 In a medium saucepan over medium heat, add the rice with the remaining 1 tablespoon of olive oil. Cook, stirring constantly, for around 4 minutes or until slightly fragrant.

4 To the rice, add ¼ cup of the pesto along with the water and balsamic vinegar. Cook on high heat and bring to a boil; then reduce to a simmer. Cover with a lid and cook for around 15 minutes, until the moisture is absorbed. Remove from the heat.

5 Stir the remaining 2 teaspoons of lemon juice and the remaining ¼ teaspoon of salt into the cooked rice. Replace the lid and allow to sit for about 5 minutes.

6 Using bamboo skewers, secure the pineapple, red pepper, and shrimp alternately on the skewers, with a total of 3 of each item per skewer. Arrange the skewers on a foil-covered baking sheet.

7 Spread the remaining pesto across the top of the skewers. Cook for around 10 minutes, until the shrimp is cooked and the pepper is slightly soft. Finish by broiling on high for 1 to 2 minutes, until slightly browned.

8 Serve the skewers on top of the pesto rice.

PER SERVING: *Calories 578 (From Fat 324); Fat 32g (Saturated 5g); Cholesterol 69mg; Sodium 613mg; Carbohydrate 57g (Dietary Fiber 5g); Protein 18g.*

NOTE: These skewers also taste delicious when grilled on the barbeque. If you choose this method, soak the wooden skewers in water for 30 minutes or more before skewering the food.

Miso Soba Noodles with Salmon

PREP TIME: 5 MIN	COOK TIME: 15 MIN	YIELD: 4 SERVINGS

INGREDIENTS

One 12-ounce (350 g) salmon fillet, skin on

⅓ cup (80 mL) plain coconut-based yogurt

3 tablespoons (45 mL) olive oil

2 tablespoons (30 mL) rice vinegar

2 tablespoons (30 mL) tamari (gluten-free)

2 tablespoons (30 mL) red or white miso

2 tablespoons (30 mL) maple syrup

1 tablespoon (15 mL) Dijon mustard

10 ounces (300 g) 100 percent buckwheat soba

1 cup (250 mL) frozen edamame beans, shelled

DIRECTIONS

1 Preheat the oven to 425°F (220°C).

2 Line a baking sheet with parchment. Place the salmon, skin down, on the prepared sheet. Bake for 10 to 12 minutes, or until the thickest part of the salmon can be flaked apart using a fork. Remove from the oven.

3 While the salmon is baking, in a small saucepan combine the yogurt, olive oil, rice vinegar, soy sauce, miso, maple syrup, and mustard. Place the saucepan on the stove over medium heat. Bring to a boil and allow the mixture to bubble for 1 minute. Remove from the heat and set aside.

4 Fill a medium pot with water and bring to a boil. Add the soba and cook for around 4 minutes or until the noodles are almost tender. Add the edamame to the pot and boil for an additional 1 minute.

5 Drain the noodles and edamame, rinse in cold water, and return to the pot. Pour the miso sauce over the top and toss to combine.

6 Divide the noodles into bowls. Flake the salmon off the skin in chunks and distribute it on top of the noodle bowls. Serve immediately.

PER SERVING: *Calories 545 (From Fat 146); Fat 16g (Saturated 3g); Cholesterol 45mg; Sodium 1300mg; Carbohydrate 69g (Dietary Fiber 3g); Protein 36g.*

NOTE: Some Dijon mustards contain onion and garlic, so check the ingredients before choosing a product to use in your low-FODMAP recipes.

NOTE: This dish provides four servings, which keeps the amount of miso per serving under the low-FODMAP limit. Remember to set your portion sizes accordingly.

Ginger Tofu Noodle Bowls

PREP TIME: 10 MIN | COOK TIME: 5 MIN | YIELD: 4 SERVINGS

INGREDIENTS

4 nests (200 g) uncooked rice noodles

2 tablespoons (30 mL) fish sauce

2 tablespoons (30 mL) soy sauce

2 tablespoons (30 mL) rice vinegar

2 teaspoons (10 mL) brown sugar

2 teaspoons (10 mL) ginger, finely chopped

2 tablespoons (30 mL) garlic-infused olive oil

1 block (350 g) extra-firm tofu, cubed

1 cup (250 mL) carrot, peeled and shredded

1 cup (250 mL) green pepper, finely chopped

2 tablespoons (30 mL) green onion tops, finely chopped

1 cup (250 mL) bean sprouts

2 tablespoons (30 mL) peanuts, finely chopped

DIRECTIONS

1 Place the rice noodles in a large bowl and cover with boiling water. Let stand for 3 minutes. Then drain, rinse with cold water, and set aside.

2 In a small bowl, combine the fish sauce, soy sauce, rice vinegar, brown sugar, and ginger. Mix well.

3 In a medium skillet over medium–high heat, add the olive oil and the tofu. Fry the tofu for around 3 minutes, until slightly browned.

4 Add around half of the prepared sauce to the skillet with the tofu; then add the carrot and green pepper. Fry for around 1 minute, until the vegetables are slightly softened. Remove from the heat and stir in the green onion tops.

5 Divide the noodles into 2 bowls. Top each bowl with half of the tofu mixture; then divide the remaining sauce between the bowls. Garnish with the bean sprouts and crushed peanuts. Serve immediately.

PER SERVING: *Calories 386 (From Fat 101); Fat 11g (Saturated 2g); Cholesterol 0mg; Sodium 1394mg; Carbohydrate 59g (Dietary Fiber 3g); Protein 12g.*

NOTE: Tofu is low-FODMAP as long as you use firm or extra-firm varieties.

TIP: To make this dish vegetarian, substitute tamari for the specified amount of fish sauce.

Sweet-and-Sour Pineapple Fish

PREP TIME: 5 MIN	COOK TIME: 15 MIN	YIELD: 4 SERVINGS

INGREDIENTS

3 cups (750 mL) water

1½ cups (375 mL) uncooked rice

Two 10-ounce (280 g) fillets of halibut or other firm fish (such as tilapia)

4 tablespoons (60 mL) plus ½ cup (125 mL) pineapple juice, divided

2 tablespoons (30 mL) cornstarch

4 tablespoons (60 mL) brown sugar

2 tablespoons (30 mL) white vinegar

2 teaspoons (10 mL) soy sauce

4 teaspoons (20 mL) tomato paste

2 tablespoons (30 mL) canned crushed pineapple, drained

DIRECTIONS

1 Preheat the oven to 425°F (220°C).

2 In a medium pot, bring the water to a boil over medium-high heat. Add the rice and return to a boil, stirring once. Reduce the heat to low and cover the pot, continuing to cook on low for 20 minutes. Remove from the heat and keep covered.

3 Line a baking sheet with parchment. Place the fish on the prepared sheet of parchment. Bake for 12 to 15 minutes, or until the thickest part of the fish can be flaked apart using a fork. Remove from the oven.

4 In a small saucepan, whisk together 2 tablespoons of the pineapple juice and the cornstarch until no lumps remain.

5 Turn the saucepan heat to medium and add the remaining ¼ cup of pineapple juice along with the brown sugar, white vinegar, soy sauce, tomato paste, and crushed pineapple. Stirring continually, heat until the mixture starts to bubble. Remove from the heat.

6 Flake apart the fish into 1-inch chunks and add to the sauce. Mix gently.

7 Serve over the rice or another grain of your choice.

PER SERVING: *Calories 466 (From Fat 20); Fat 2g (Saturated 1g); Cholesterol 68mg; Sodium 294mg; Carbohydrate 76g (Dietary Fiber 1g); Protein 32g.*

Cooking Meat-Based Dishes with Low-FODMAP Ingredients

If you're an omnivore, you may enjoy a hearty dinner that includes some kind of meat. Beef, pork, chicken, and other meats are fine on the low–FODMAP diet — but remember that it's best to eat red meats in moderation. Chicken is a good alternative to red meat; a significant amount of research suggests that swapping out red meat and replacing it with chicken can improve health over the long term.

Here are the meat-based main dishes described in this section:

>> **Pork and Cabbage Rice-Paper Wraps:** These crispy wraps are packed with flavor from ginger, sesame oil, soy sauce, and more.

>> **Chicken and Feta Patties:** These protein-rich bites are a delicious way to use leftover cooked rice.

>> **Lemony Kale Chicken:** This meal is tasty and bright, and it takes only a few minutes to make.

>> **Chicken and Broccoli in Creamy Peanut Sauce:** This meal's creamy sauce is rich and satisfying — and it's loved by kids and adults alike.

Pork and Cabbage Rice-Paper Wraps

PREP TIME: 10 MIN	COOK TIME: 20 MIN	YIELD: 4 SERVINGS (8 WRAPS)

INGREDIENTS

1 tablespoon (15 mL) sesame oil

1 pound (450 g) ground pork

1 teaspoon (5 mL) salt

1 teaspoon (5 mL) ginger, finely chopped

2 cups (500 mL) Napa cabbage

1 cup (250 mL) carrot, peeled and shredded

1 tablespoon (15 mL) soy sauce

1 teaspoon (5 mL) white sugar

1 tablespoon (15 mL) green onion tops, finely chopped

8 dry rice-paper wraps

1 teaspoon (5 mL) olive oil (garlic-infused if desired)

2 tablespoons tamari (gluten-free)

2 tablespoons rice vinegar

Pinch of grated ginger

DIRECTIONS

1 Over medium-high heat in a large skillet, add the sesame oil, ground pork, and salt. Cook until no pink remains in the pork, around 5 to 8 minutes.

2 Add the ginger, cabbage, carrot, soy sauce, and sugar to the skillet. Cook for around 4 to 5 minutes, until the cabbage and carrot are softened. Remove from the heat.

3 Stir in the green onion tops; then pour the mixture into a colander to drain any excess moisture.

4 Prepare one of the rice wraps according to the package directions by immersing in boiled water.

5 Lay the prepared wrap on a paper towel. Put approximately ½ cup of the pork mixture in the center and wrap, folding in the sides and then rolling into a tight bundle.

6 Turn the skillet to high heat and add the olive oil. Place each wrap edge-down in the pan and cook for about 1 minute on each side, or until the wrap is slightly browned and crispy. Prepare and cook the remaining wraps.

7 In a small bowl, combine the tamari, rice vinegar, and grated ginger and mix. Use as a dipping sauce for the finished wraps.

PER SERVING: *Calories 350 (From Fat 248); Fat 28g (Saturated 9g); Cholesterol 82mg; Sodium 1190mg; Carbohydrate 4g (Dietary Fiber 1g); Protein 21g.*

TIP: If you don't have rice-paper wraps, you can serve the filling over rice for a meal in itself. If you're using wraps, fry only the number of wraps you currently need, and store the remaining filling in the fridge.

Chicken and Feta Patties

PREP TIME: 5 MIN	COOK TIME: 15 MIN	YIELD: 4 SERVINGS (12 SMALL PATTIES)

INGREDIENTS

1 pound (450 g) ground chicken

½ cup (125 mL) white rice, cooked

¼ cup (60 mL) feta cheese, crumbled

½ teaspoon (2.5 mL) salt

Pinch of ground pepper

1 egg

½ teaspoon (2.5 mL) dried oregano

½ cup (125 mL) water, divided

1 tablespoon (15 g) extra-virgin olive oil, divided

Balsamic vinegar for garnish (optional)

DIRECTIONS

1 In a medium bowl, combine the chicken, rice, feta cheese, salt, pepper, egg, and oregano. Mix well.

2 Shape the mixture into 12 small patties and arrange on a plate or a sheet of parchment.

3 In a large frying pan over medium heat, add ¼ cup of the water and ½ tablespoon of the olive oil. When heated, place 6 patties in the frying pan. Cook for approximately 5 minutes on each side. When the water is evaporated, cook for an additional 2 to 3 minutes on each side until lightly browned. Remove the patties from the frying pan.

4 Add the remaining ¼ cup of water and the remaining ½ tablespoon of olive oil to the frying pan and cook the remaining patties the same way. Keep the cooked patties warm until it's time to serve. Drizzle with balsamic vinegar if desired.

PER SERVING: *Calories 246 (From Fat 132); Fat 15g (Saturated 4g); Cholesterol 106mg; Sodium 477mg; Carbohydrate 6g (Dietary Fiber 0g); Protein 23g.*

Lemony Kale Chicken

PREP TIME: 5 MIN | COOK TIME: 20 MIN | YIELD: 4 SERVINGS

INGREDIENTS

3 cups (750 mL) water

1½ cups (375 mL) uncooked rice

4 tablespoons (60 mL) pine nuts

4 tablespoons (60 mL) garlic-infused olive oil, divided

4 chicken breasts, cut into bite-size pieces

4 cups (1 L) curly green kale, destemmed and chopped

2 teaspoons (10 mL) salt

Pinch of black pepper

4 teaspoons (20 mL) lemon zest

4 tablespoons (60 mL) lemon juice

2 tablespoons (30 mL) brown sugar

1 teaspoon (5 mL) smoked paprika

DIRECTIONS

1 In a medium pot, bring the water to a boil over medium-high heat. Add the rice and return to a boil, stirring once. Reduce the heat to low and cover the pot, continuing to cook on low for 20 minutes. Remove from the heat and keep covered.

2 In a small frying pan over medium-high heat, toast the pine nuts for 1 to 2 minutes, stirring continually until lightly browned. Set aside.

3 In a large skillet over medium-high heat, add 2 tablespoons of the olive oil and cook the chicken for approximately 8 to 10 minutes or until cooked through and slightly browned.

4 Add the kale to the skillet and cook for around 3 minutes or until softened.

5 Reduce the skillet heat to medium. In a small bowl, combine the salt, pepper, lemon zest, the remaining 2 tablespoons of olive oil, lemon juice, brown sugar, and paprika and mix. Add the sauce to the skillet and simmer until the flavors are combined, around 2 minutes.

6 Serve over the rice or another grain of your choice. Garnish with the toasted pine nuts.

PER SERVING: *Calories 581 (From Fat 199); Fat 22g (Saturated 22g); Cholesterol 47mg; Sodium 1419mg; Carbohydrate 70g (Dietary Fiber 3g); Protein 26g.*

Chicken and Broccoli in Creamy Peanut Sauce

PREP TIME: 5 MIN	COOK TIME: 30 MIN	YIELD: 4 SERVINGS

INGREDIENTS

3 cups (750 mL) water

1½ cups (375 mL) uncooked rice

1 teaspoon (5 mL) garlic-infused olive oil

4 chicken breasts, cut into bite-size pieces

¼ cup (60 mL) salted natural peanut butter, smooth

1 tablespoon (15 mL) brown sugar

3 tablespoons (45 mL) soy sauce

1 can (400 mL) coconut milk

2 cups (500 mL) broccoli florets, destemmed (around 1 medium crown)

DIRECTIONS

1 In a medium pot, bring the water to a boil over medium-high heat. Add the rice and return to a boil, stirring once. Reduce the heat to low and cover the pot, continuing to cook on low for 20 minutes. Remove from the heat and keep covered.

2 In a large skillet over medium-high heat, warm the olive oil. Add the chicken and fry until cooked through and slightly browned, around 8 to 10 minutes.

3 In a medium bowl, stir together the peanut butter, brown sugar, and soy sauce.

4 After the chicken is cooked, reduce the skillet heat to medium. Pour in the coconut milk.

5 Add the peanut butter mixture to the skillet and gently stir. Continue to stir for 5 to 6 minutes until the mixture is brought to a simmer.

6 Add the broccoli florets and continue to simmer for 5 to 6 minutes until the broccoli is slightly tender. Serve over the rice or another grain of your choice.

PER SERVING: *Calories 654 (From Fat 270); Fat 30g (Saturated 19g); Cholesterol 47mg; Sodium 1080mg; Carbohydrate 68g (Dietary Fiber 3g); Protein 31g.*

TIP: If you prefer a meat-free version of this dish, you can substitute the chicken with cubes of firm or extra-firm tofu, lightly fried. Three-quarters of a cup of broccoli per person is considered a low-FODMAP portion.

Chapter 20

Sides and Snacks

The low–FODMAP diet may mean eliminating some of the foods you normally would've eaten, which means every bite counts for gaining valuable nutrients. Each side dish and snack is an opportunity to pack in more nutrition to keep your body healthy and strong. Foods such as potato chips and french fries, though technically allowed on a low-FODMAP diet, should be a last resort because you need to fill your belly with a variety of foods that help you meet your daily nutritional needs.

TECHNICAL STUFF

FODMAP stands for *fermentable oligosaccharides, disaccharides, monosaccharides and polyols.* Read more about a low–FODMAP diet in Chapter 8.

In this chapter, we provide recipes for side dishes as well as snacks and appetizers that will sustain you with valuable nutrients and make your taste buds happy, too. First, you find four tasty low–FODMAP side dishes; then you find some flavorful choices for snacks and appetizers that are designed to avoiding triggering troublesome gut symptoms.

Enjoying Gut-Friendly Side Dishes

In the same way that a good pair of shoes really sets off an outfit, a good side dish elevates a main meal and showcases its best qualities. This section gives you an array of interesting low-FODMAP side dishes that pack a nutritional punch.

The following recipes are found in this section:

>> **Parmesan Quinoa Patties:** These savory patties will soon become a household favorite. They pair well with herbed, grilled chicken.

>> **Cheesy Waffles:** Give your waffle maker new life with these super-easy crispy cheese waffles.

>> **Dill Zucchini Rounds:** These zucchini rounds have the taste of dill pickle chips, but with a lot more vitamins. They're the perfect accompaniment to grilled fish or meat.

>> **Savory Green Onion Pancakes:** These tasty pancakes, made with FODMAP-friendly green onion tops, are great on their own as a snack or eaten with a main meal to soak up the juices of a stir-fry.

Parmesan Quinoa Patties

PREP TIME: 5 MIN	COOK TIME: 40 MIN	YIELD: 4 SERVINGS (8 PATTIES)

INGREDIENTS

1 cup (250 mL) uncooked quinoa

2 cups (500 mL) water

1 tablespoon (15 mL) basil leaves, finely chopped

1 tablespoon (15 mL) oregano leaves, finely chopped

½ teaspoon (2.5 mL) salt

2 eggs, lightly beaten

¼ cup (60 mL) grated Parmesan cheese

½ cup (125 mL) quick oats

1 tablespoon (15 mL) extra-virgin olive oil

DIRECTIONS

1 In a medium saucepan over medium-high heat, combine the quinoa and water. Bring to a boil; then reduce the heat to medium and simmer for around 15 minutes, stirring occasionally, until the water is absorbed. Remove from the heat; then cover and let the quinoa sit for 10 minutes.

2 In a large bowl, combine 1 cup of the cooked quinoa with the basil, oregano, salt, eggs, Parmesan cheese, and oats. Mix well.

3 Shape the mixture into 8 small patties and place on a parchment-covered plate. Refrigerate for 10 to 15 minutes.

4 In a medium skillet, heat the olive oil over medium-high heat. Fry the patties for 3 to 5 minutes on each side, or until lightly browned. Serve immediately.

PER SERVING: *Calories 286 (From Fat 98); Fat 11g (Saturated 3g); Cholesterol 111mg; Sodium 424mg; Carbohydrate 35g (Dietary Fiber 4g); Protein 13g.*

NOTE: This recipe also works well with leftover plain quinoa from the fridge — if you have some, skip Step 1.

TIP: In place of water, you can use a homemade vegetable-based broth or chicken broth made without garlic and onion. See the Chapter 18 sidebar "The low-FODMAP broth problem."

Cheesy Waffles

| PREP TIME: 5 MIN | COOK TIME: 5 MIN | YIELD: 4 SERVINGS |

INGREDIENTS

2 cups (500 mL) Gruyère cheese, grated

2 cups (500 mL) white cheddar cheese, grated

8 eggs

½ cup (125 mL) coconut flour

2 teaspoons (10 mL) baking powder

Pinch of black pepper

DIRECTIONS

1 Preheat a waffle maker to medium heat.

2 In a medium bowl, combine all the ingredients. Mix well.

3 Pour half of the mixture into the waffle maker and spread gently before closing the iron.

4 When indicated by the ready light (around 5 minutes), remove the waffle from the waffle maker. Repeat to make additional waffles. Serve immediately.

PER SERVING: *Calories 655 (From Fat 433); Fat 48g (Saturated 27g); Cholesterol 542mg; Sodium 926mg; Carbohydrate 10g (Dietary Fiber 6g); Protein 45g.*

NOTE: This savory waffle tastes great with fresh, flavorful toppings (for example, arugula, prosciutto, and shredded mozzarella cheese with a vinaigrette dressing drizzled on top).

Dill Zucchini Rounds

PREP TIME: 5 MIN   COOK TIME: 1 HR   YIELD: 4 SERVINGS

INGREDIENTS

1⅓ medium zucchini (or ½ large zucchini), thinly sliced

2 tablespoons (30 mL) extra-virgin olive oil

½ teaspoon (2.5 mL) salt

2 tablespoons (30 mL) white vinegar

½ teaspoon (2.5 mL) Dijon mustard

1 teaspoon (5 mL) dried dill

1 teaspoon (5 mL) dried basil

1 teaspoon (5 mL) lemon juice

DIRECTIONS

1 Preheat the oven to 325°F (160°C).

2 Line a baking sheet with parchment.

3 Blot each zucchini round with a paper towel; then transfer to a medium bowl.

4 In small bowl, combine the olive oil, salt, vinegar, mustard, dill, basil, and lemon juice.

5 Reserve 2 tablespoons of the dressing. Pour the rest of the dressing over the zucchini rounds and toss to coat.

6 Arrange the rounds on the prepared baking sheet. Bake for 30 minutes; then remove from the oven and flip the zucchini rounds before baking for an additional 30 minutes. The zucchini rounds should be brown and slightly curled at the edges. Toss with the reserved dressing. Serve hot or cold.

PER SERVING: *Calories 71 (From Fat 63); Fat 7g (Saturated 1g); Cholesterol 0mg; Sodium 296mg; Carbohydrate 2g (Dietary Fiber 1g); Protein 1g.*

Savory Green Onion Pancakes

INGREDIENTS

½ cup (125 mL) almond flour

1 cup (250 mL) rice flour

1 teaspoon (5 mL) baking soda

1 teaspoon (5 mL) salt

2 teaspoons (10 mL)
white sugar

1 cup (250 mL) water

2 eggs

4 tablespoons (60 mL)
butter, melted

4 tablespoons (60 mL) green
onion tops, finely chopped

2 teaspoons (10 mL) sesame oil

2 tablespoons tamari
(gluten-free)

2 tablespoons rice vinegar

Pinch of grated ginger

DIRECTIONS

1 In a large bowl, mix the almond flour, rice flour, baking soda, salt, and sugar. Stir well to combine.

2 Add the water, egg, and melted butter, and stir until the mixture is a smooth consistency. Add the green onion tops and mix.

3 Heat the sesame oil in a small frying pan over medium–high heat. Pour half of the batter into the frying pan and cook the pancake for about 3 minutes per side, or until browned. Repeat with the remaining batter.

4 In a small bowl, combine the tamari, rice vinegar, and grated ginger and mix. Use as a dipping sauce for the hot or cold pancakes.

PER SERVING: *Calories 398 (From Fat 215); Fat 24g (Saturated 9g); Cholesterol 136mg; Sodium 1202mg; Carbohydrate 38g (Dietary Fiber 3g); Protein 10g.*

Supporting Your Digestion with Tasty Snacks and Appetizers

The best approach to snacking, whether you have irritable bowel syndrome (IBS) or not, is the classic Boy Scout motto: Be prepared. When you have an extended period of time between meals and you know you'll be hungry, plan ahead so you'll be able to make good snacking choices and avoid irritating your belly. Make a habit of carrying extra IBS-friendly snacks in your bag when you go out: carrot sticks, a hard-boiled egg, plain popcorn, or another food you know you can tolerate.

The same preparedness maxim goes for appetizers. If you're attending a dinner party, for example, a lot of unknowns may exist, including the timing of the meal and whether you'll have options for foods you can tolerate. If you bring a tasty low-FODMAP appetizer to share with others before the meal, you'll be able to stave off your own hunger while doing the host a favor.

Here are the snacks and appetizers detailed in this section:

>> **Roasted Carrot Dip:** This delicious dip is great for veggies or low-FODMAP crackers. It also makes a great spread for sandwiches that use low-FODMAP bread.

>> **Bacon-Wrapped Water Chestnuts:** Be prepared to be the most popular person at the potluck if you bring these. They're rich and satisfying with the bacon and caramelized sugar.

>> **Herb and Tomato Polenta Rounds:** These rounds make an eye-catching appetizer, or try them for a light lunch.

>> **Chicken Meatballs with Sweet Orange Sauce:** Kids and adults alike will love these easy and tasty chicken meatballs.

>> **Deluxe Deviled Eggs:** The addition of flavorful smoked salmon creates a twist on the classic deviled egg.

SNACKING WHEN YOU HAVE IBS

The influence of snacking on IBS can vary from person to person, but in general, smaller meals and snacks are less likely to set off gut symptoms than large meals (especially high-fat ones). Spacing your meals and snacks three hours apart can be helpful, because this allows the muscles of the digestive tract enough time to sweep the food through your digestive tract from the stomach to the large intestine. If you snack too frequently, you prevent the sweeping motion from occurring, which can lead to IBS symptoms.

As simple as it sounds, slowing down your eating and chewing your food well is important in IBS. Whether you're having a full meal or a snack, take the time to sit down, free of distractions (including phones and tablets), and focus on enjoying your food. It's amazing what a difference a mindful eating pattern can make.

Snacking with IBS doesn't have to be complicated or time-consuming. Here are some ideas for quick and easy snacks that require minimal preparation:

- **Protein:** Hard-boiled egg with sea salt, hard cheese, nut butter, nuts without sugar or salt, tuna

- **Fruits:** Banana, cantaloupe melon (a small portion), kiwi, orange, pineapple

- **Vegetables:** Carrots, red pepper (a small portion)

- **Grains:** Gluten-free or low-FODMAP crackers, popcorn, rice cakes, rice crackers

Roasted Carrot Dip

PREP TIME: 10 MIN	COOK TIME: 30 MIN	YIELD: 4 SERVINGS

INGREDIENTS

6 medium carrots, peeled and chopped into approximately 2-inch chunks

1 tablespoon (15 mL) extra-virgin olive oil (garlic-infused, if desired)

½ teaspoon (2.5 mL) salt

¼ cup (60 g) plain goat cheese

1 tablespoon (15 mL) lemon juice

1 tablespoon (15 mL) maple syrup

Pinch of black pepper

Chili flakes for garnish (optional)

Additional olive oil for garnish (optional)

DIRECTIONS

1 Preheat the oven to 425°F (220°C).

2 Line a baking sheet with parchment. Arrange the carrots in a single layer on the prepared sheet and drizzle with the olive oil and salt. Toss gently.

3 Roast for 20 minutes; then remove from the oven and toss. Return to the oven for another 10 to 15 minutes, until the carrots are fork-tender and lightly browned.

4 Cool the carrots slightly; then place them in a blender (or bowl if using an immersion blender) with the goat cheese, lemon juice, maple syrup, and pepper. Blend until smooth.

5 Spread out the dip onto a plate or serving board. Garnish with the chili flakes and a drizzle of olive oil if desired.

PER SERVING: *Calories 113 (From Fat 55); Fat 6g (Saturated 2g); Cholesterol 7mg; Sodium 390mg; Carbohydrate 13g (Dietary Fiber 3g); Protein 3g.*

TIP: Serve with veggie sticks or low-FODMAP crackers. Rice crackers, rice cakes, and rye crackers (such as Wasa Crispbread, with a portion size of 1 large cracker) are good options.

Bacon-Wrapped Water Chestnuts

PREP TIME: 5 MIN | COOK TIME: 25 MIN | YIELD: 4 SERVINGS (12 PIECES)

INGREDIENTS

¼ cup (60 mL) soy sauce

One 8-ounce (227 mL) can whole water chestnuts, drained

¼ cup (60 mL) brown sugar

6 strips of uncooked smoked bacon

DIRECTIONS

1 Preheat the oven to 400°F (200°C).

2 Place the soy sauce in a medium bowl and add the water chestnuts. Marinate in the refrigerator for 1 hour.

3 Line a baking sheet with foil.

4 Cut each strip of bacon in half.

5 Add the brown sugar to a small bowl. Roll each water chestnut in the brown sugar; then wrap it in half a strip of bacon. Secure with a toothpick on top and place on the prepared baking sheet.

6 Bake for 25 minutes, or until the bacon is browned and bubbling. Serve hot or cold.

PER SERVING: *Calories 142 (From Fat 45); Fat 5g (Saturated 2g); Cholesterol 13mg; Sodium 542mg; Carbohydrate 19g (Dietary Fiber 2g); Protein 5g.*

Herb and Tomato Polenta Rounds

PREP TIME: 5 MIN	COOK TIME: 15 MIN	YIELD: 4 SERVINGS (12 PIECES)

INGREDIENTS

½ tube (340 g) ready-to-eat polenta

1 tablespoon (15 mL) olive oil

One 4-ounce package (113 g) plain goat cheese

¼ teaspoon (1 mL) salt

Pinch of black pepper

¼ teaspoon (1 mL) dried rosemary

1 teaspoon (5 mL) dried basil

1 tablespoon (15 mL) lactose-free milk

12 cherry tomatoes, cut into rounds

DIRECTIONS

1 Slice the polenta into 12 thin rounds, approximately ¼ inch (0.5 cm) thick.

2 Heat the olive oil in a large skillet over medium-high heat. Add a layer of polenta rounds and fry for around 4 minutes on each side until slightly browned.

3 Transfer the rounds to a paper-towel-lined plate.

4 In a medium bowl, combine the goat cheese, salt, pepper, rosemary, and basil. Mix well with a fork. Add the milk and stir until evenly thinned.

5 Spread a layer of the goat cheese mixture onto each polenta round and top with several slices of cherry tomato.

6 Broil the rounds in the oven (around 8 inches or 20 cm from the burner) on high for approximately 3 minutes, until the tomatoes soften and release their juices. Serve warm or cold.

PER SERVING: *Calories 228 (From Fat 110); Fat 12g (Saturated 6g); Cholesterol 22mg; Sodium 465mg; Carbohydrate 21g (Dietary Fiber 2g); Protein 9g.*

Chicken Meatballs with Sweet Orange Sauce

PREP TIME: 10 MIN	COOK TIME: 20 MIN	YIELD: 4 SERVINGS (12 MEATBALLS)

INGREDIENTS

1 pound (500 g) uncooked ground chicken

⅔ cup (170 mL) quick oats

½ teaspoon (2.5 mL) salt

Pinch of black pepper

1 egg, slightly beaten

1 tablespoon (15 mL) sesame seeds

3 tablespoons (45 mL) cold water

2 tablespoons (30 mL) orange juice

1 teaspoon (5 mL) cornstarch

1 tablespoon (15 mL) soy sauce

2 tablespoons (30 mL) brown sugar

1½ teaspoons (7.5 mL) orange zest

DIRECTIONS

1 Preheat the oven to 400°F (200°C).

2 Place the ground chicken in a large bowl and add the oats, salt, pepper, and egg. Mix well.

3 Line a baking sheet with parchment. Place mounds of the chicken mixture (approximately 2 tablespoons each, shaped into balls) onto the prepared sheet and bake for approximately 20 minutes, or until cooked through with an internal temperature of 165 °F (75°C).

4 Turn the oven to broil (on high) for about 3 minutes or until the tops of the meatballs are slightly browned.

5 While the meatballs are baking, place the sesame seeds in a small frying pan over medium-high heat. Toast for about 1 minute, stirring constantly, until slightly browned. Set aside.

6 In a small saucepan, combine the water and orange juice. Add the cornstarch, and whisk until smooth.

7 Turn the heat to medium and add the soy sauce, brown sugar, and orange zest. Stir until the mixture thickens and starts to bubble, around 3 to 4 minutes. Remove from the heat.

8 When the meatballs are done cooking, transfer them to a serving dish. Pour the sauce over the top and sprinkle with sesame seeds. Serve immediately.

PER SERVING: *Calories 254 (From Fat 103); Fat 11g (Saturated 3g); Cholesterol 105mg; Sodium 804mg; Carbohydrate 17g (Dietary Fiber 2g); Protein 21g.*

Deluxe Deviled Eggs

PREP TIME: 10 MIN	COOK TIME: 20 MIN	YIELD: 4 SERVINGS

INGREDIENTS

6 eggs

1 teaspoon (5 mL) apple cider vinegar

1 teaspoon (5 mL) yellow mustard

½ teaspoon (2.5 mL) dried dill

2 tablespoons (30 mL) mayonnaise

Pinch of salt

Pinch of black pepper

2 tablespoons (30 mL) smoked salmon, finely chopped

2 teaspoons (10 mL) green onion tops, finely chopped

DIRECTIONS

1 Place the eggs in a medium pot and cover with cold water.

2 Heat the pot on the stovetop on high heat. When the water reaches a boil, wait 1 minute and then remove from the heat. Let stand for 15 minutes.

3 Drain the water off the eggs and rinse in cold water. When cooled, carefully peel the shells off the eggs.

4 Cut the eggs in half and gently remove the yolks. Arrange the halves on a plate, rounded side down.

5 Place the yolks in a medium bowl and add the apple cider vinegar, mustard, dill, mayonnaise, salt, pepper, salmon, and green onion tops. Mash together and stir until well combined.

6 Spoon the mixture into the egg halves. Chill in the refrigerator, covered, until ready to serve.

PER SERVING: *Calories 145 (From Fat 92); Fat 10g (Saturated 3g); Cholesterol 321mg; Sodium 266mg; Carbohydrate 2g (Dietary Fiber 0g); Protein 11g.*

NOTE: In the place of smoked salmon and green onion tops, you can try different flavorful combinations such as lemon juice and dill or basil.

Chapter **21**

Desserts

Although healthy diet patterns such as the Mediterranean diet incorporate very few sweets, the truth is that sweet foods are almost universally appealing and they can be one of life's simple pleasures. Rest assured, sweets can definitely be a part of a well-rounded diet that benefits your health. Consuming sweets in moderation is perfectly fine and may even prevent you from bingeing (for example, eating an entire tub of ice cream) when you let down your guard.

The sugar used in baked items and desserts is generally not a problem for the low-FODMAP diet used for irritable bowel syndrome (IBS), because these simple sugars are absorbed in the digestive tract before reaching the large intestine (which is where the troublesome nonabsorbable sugars can cause symptoms). But many sweets that are common in North America and Europe contain other gut-irritating ingredients — most commonly, wheat flour.

TECHNICAL STUFF

FODMAP stands for *fermentable oligosaccharides, disaccharides, monosaccharides and polyols*. Read more about a low-FODMAP diet in Chapter 8.

The key to incorporating sweets into a healthy diet is choosing the right ones: preferably the sweets you make yourself, rather than the ultra-processed, sugar-loaded sweets that line the grocery store shelves.

This chapter gives you inspiration for making your own delicious sweets, with recipes designed to deliver some nutritional value beyond the quick-burning sugars. It's a great idea to make some of these items and store them in the fridge or freezer so you have something to grab that's friendly to your digestion when you feel like having a little dose of sugar.

REMEMBER

All desserts, even the ones in this chapter, should be consumed in moderation. Some of the recipes in this chapter contain FODMAPs in low amounts, which shouldn't bother you if eaten in the proper serving sizes. But if you indulge in more than one serving per sitting, it may push your FODMAP intake over the limit and cause digestive symptoms.

In this chapter, you find recipes for low-FODMAP sweets that are both tasty and satisfying. The first section of the chapter features snacks you can make and take with you out of the house, and the next section shares fruit-focused desserts for something special after a meal.

Baking Snacks to Grab and Go

Baking is a new adventure when you adopt a low-FODMAP diet. You can't rely on some of the traditional baking ingredients, such as wheat flour and milk, but you can still create delicious treats with a little out-of-the-box thinking.

The recipes in this section are examples of how you can use low-FODMAP ingredients to bake batches of items suitable for taking with you out of the house. When you have some of these on hand, you may not be as tempted to indulge in some of the store-bought sweets that will bother your digestion later on.

The following recipes are found in this section:

>> **Carrot Cake Bites:** Super soft and moist, these delicious morsels taste remarkably similar to carrot cake but require zero baking.

>> **Chocolate Coconut Power Cookies:** These cookies are chewy and satisfying any time of the day — and with loads of oats and coconut, they make a great breakfast.

>> **Chocolate Chip Chia Energy Balls:** These dense energy balls are a filling snack to have on hand for after school or work. They also taste amazing as a quick breakfast paired with a black coffee.

>> **Pumpkin Spice Oatmeal Muffins:** These muffins (or more accurately, muffin tops) are delicious and decadent with their mixture of warm spices and chocolate chips.

SUCCESSFUL LOW-FODMAP BAKING

When you're on a low-FODMAP diet, suitable premade baked goods are very hard to come by. Homemade baking is the best way to go. However, simply substituting low-FODMAP ingredients into a regular recipe may yield unpredictable results because of the properties of the flour and other ingredients. When you're making a batch of low-FODMAP baked items, try to use an IBS-friendly recipe someone else has already tested.

Many gluten-free flours are also low-FODMAP but be sure to double-check the FODMAP content of any gluten-free flour before using it. Here are some low-FODMAP flours you may consider using in your baking:

- Buckwheat flour
- Maize or corn flour
- Millet flour
- Oat flour
- Quinoa flour
- Rice flour

Many sugars are okay to use in your baking on a low-FODMAP diet. Honey in large amounts is not low-FODMAP, but most other types of sugar are okay to use as long as they don't specifically trigger your gut symptoms. Some sugars that are allowed (in reasonable amounts, of course) on a low-FODMAP diet are as follows:

- Brown sugar
- Icing sugar
- Maple syrup
- Palm sugar
- White sugar

Carrot Cake Bites

PREP TIME: 15 MIN	COOK TIME: NONE	YIELD: 6 SERVINGS (12 BALLS)

INGREDIENTS

2 tablespoons (30 mL) coconut oil

¾ cup (180 mL) finely shredded carrot (approximately one medium carrot)

¼ cup (60 mL) maple syrup

½ teaspoon (2.5 mL) apple cider vinegar

1 teaspoon (5 mL) vanilla extract

½ teaspoon (2.5 mL) cinnamon

¼ teaspoon (1 mL) ground ginger

¼ teaspoon (1 mL) ground nutmeg

¼ teaspoon (1 mL) salt

1 cup (250 mL) almond flour

¼ cup (60 mL) pecans, finely chopped

2 tablespoons (30 mL) hemp seeds

¼ cup (60 mL) medium shredded coconut, unsweetened

DIRECTIONS

1 Put the coconut oil into a small microwave-safe bowl and microwave for 30 seconds or until clear. (You can also do this on the stovetop.) Set it aside while you prepare the rest of the ingredients.

2 In a large bowl, combine the shredded carrot, maple syrup, apple cider vinegar, vanilla, cinnamon, ginger, nutmeg, salt, almond flour, pecans, and hemp seeds. Stir until well combined.

3 Add the coconut oil to the other ingredients and stir well.

4 Using approximately 1 tablespoon of the mixture at a time, shape into balls. Gently roll each ball in the shredded coconut until coated. Chill in the refrigerator for at least 3 hours.

PER SERVING: *Calories 267 (From Fat 194); Fat 22g (Saturated 8g); Cholesterol 0mg; Sodium 110mg; Carbohydrate 16g (Dietary Fiber 4g); Protein 6g.*

Chocolate Coconut Power Cookies

PREP TIME: 10 MIN	COOK TIME: 12 MIN	YIELD: 9 SERVINGS (18 COOKIES)

INGREDIENTS

1 cup (250 mL) rice flour

1 cup (250 mL) rolled oats

½ cup (125 mL) shredded dried coconut, unsweetened

½ cup (125 mL) brown sugar

¼ cup (60 mL) cocoa powder

1 egg, lightly beaten

2 teaspoons (10 mL) vanilla extract

½ cup (125 mL) almond milk, unsweetened

¼ cup (60 mL) butter, melted

DIRECTIONS

1 Preheat the oven to 350°F (180°C).

2 In a large bowl, combine the flour, oats, coconut, brown sugar, and cocoa powder. Mix well.

3 In a medium bowl, combine the egg, vanilla, almond milk, and butter. Stir to combine.

4 Add the wet ingredients to the bowl of dry ingredients and mix until the consistency is even.

5 Shape into small balls and arrange on a parchment-covered cookie sheet. Press down each ball with a fork. Bake for 10 to 12 minutes.

PER SERVING: *Calories 258 (From Fat 99); Fat 11g (Saturated 7g); Cholesterol 37mg; Sodium 49mg; Carbohydrate 36g (Dietary Fiber 4g); Protein 6g.*

Chocolate Chip Chia Energy Balls

PREP TIME: 10 MIN | COOK TIME: NONE | YIELD: 6 SERVINGS (12 BALLS)

INGREDIENTS

1½ cups (375 mL) quick oats

½ cup (125 mL) icing sugar (powdered sugar)

1 tablespoon (15 mL) chia seeds

1 cup (250 mL) peanut butter

1 teaspoon (5 mL) vanilla extract

1 tablespoon (15 mL) maple syrup

2 tablespoons (30 mL) water

¼ cup (60 mL) chocolate chips

DIRECTIONS

1 In a large bowl, mix the oats, icing sugar, and chia seeds.

2 Add the peanut butter, vanilla, maple syrup, and water. Stir well to create an even consistency.

3 Add the chocolate chips and mix.

4 Shape the mixture into balls and refrigerate for at least 1 hour before serving.

PER SERVING: *Calories 420 (From Fat 233); Fat 26g (Saturated 6g); Cholesterol 0mg; Sodium 200mg; Carbohydrate 40g (Dietary Fiber 6g); Protein 14g.*

TIP: If the mixture is slightly crumbly, shaping it into balls works best with slightly wet hands.

Pumpkin Spice Oatmeal Muffins

PREP TIME: 20 MIN	COOK TIME: 30 MIN	YIELD: 6 SERVINGS (12 MUFFINS)

INGREDIENTS

2½ cups (625 mL) quick oats

1½ cups (375 mL) lactose-free milk

¾ cup (180 mL) canned pumpkin puree

½ cup (125 mL) brown sugar

1 teaspoon (5 mL) ground cinnamon

½ teaspoon (2.5 mL) ground ginger

½ teaspoon (2.5 mL) ground nutmeg

Pinch of ground cloves

2 tablespoons (30 mL) extra-virgin olive oil

1 egg

1 tablespoon (15 mL) baking powder

½ teaspoon (2.5 mL) salt

½ cup (125 mL) chocolate chips

DIRECTIONS

1 Preheat the oven to 350°F (180°C). Grease 12 muffin tins.

2 In a large bowl, combine the oats, milk, and pumpkin. Let sit for 10 minutes, allowing the oats to soak up the moisture.

3 Add the brown sugar, cinnamon, ginger, nutmeg, cloves, olive oil, egg, baking powder, and salt. Mix well.

4 Add the chocolate chips and mix.

5 Pour the batter into the muffin tins and bake for 30 minutes, or until a toothpick inserted in the center of a muffin comes out clean. Serve right away or store in a sealed container in the fridge or freezer.

PER SERVING: *Calories 339 (From Fat 127); Fat 14g (Saturated 5g); Cholesterol 44mg; Sodium 559mg; Carbohydrate 50g (Dietary Fiber 5g); Protein 9g.*

Whipping Up IBS-Friendly Desserts

Fresh fruit is a great go-to dessert when you want something sweet after a meal. And if you want something even more decadent, a prepared fruit-based dessert is a great choice. This section features five light and easy desserts with low-FODMAP fruits as the main ingredients.

Here are the desserts in this section:

» **Strawberry Chia Pudding:** With no cooking required, this dessert is easy to whip up and makes a nice, light finish to a meal.

» **Pavlovas with Raspberry Sauce:** Try this recipe featuring — feather-light meringue with a rich raspberry sauce — if you're looking for a stunning-looking dessert to impress guests.

» **Dreamy Banana Cream Dessert:** This dessert gives you the classic taste of banana cream pie without the hassle of making a traditional pie crust.

» **Caramelized Bananas:** The bananas in this recipe take on a pudding-like softness and are perfect garnished with chocolate, nuts, and a little coconut-based whipped cream.

» **Piña Colada Popsicles:** These tasty popsicles are great any time a cool, tropical twist fills the bill.

Strawberry Chia Pudding

PREP TIME: 10 MIN	COOK TIME: NONE	YIELD: 4 SERVINGS

INGREDIENTS

1½ cups (375 mL) fresh strawberries, hulled and diced

¼ cup (60 mL) chia seeds

1 cup (250 mL) canned coconut milk

1 tablespoon (15 mL) white sugar

Fresh strawberries for garnish

DIRECTIONS

1 In a medium bowl, combine the strawberries with the chia seeds, coconut milk, and sugar.

2 Blend the mixture lightly using an immersion blender. Some larger chunks of strawberry may remain.

3 Place the mixture in the fridge for 15 minutes.

4 Remove from the fridge, stir, and divide into 4 individual serving bowls.

5 Return the bowls to the fridge for at least 15 more minutes. Garnish with a fresh strawberry if desired and serve.

PER SERVING: *Calories 210 (From Fat 149); Fat 17g (Saturated 11g); Cholesterol 0mg; Sodium 11mg; Carbohydrate 15g (Dietary Fiber 6g); Protein 4g.*

Pavlovas with Raspberry Sauce

PREP TIME: 15 MIN	COOK TIME: 45 MIN	YIELD: 4 SERVINGS

INGREDIENTS

2 egg whites, at room temperature

Pinch of cream of tartar

½ cup (125 mL) plus 1 tablespoon (15 mL) white sugar, divided

1 cup (250 mL) fresh or frozen raspberries

¼ cup (60 mL) water

½ teaspoon (2.5 mL) orange zest

4 to 8 mint leaves for garnish (optional)

Fresh raspberries or other low-FODMAP berries for garnish (optional)

Coconut-based whipped cream for garnish (optional)

DIRECTIONS

1 Preheat the oven to 200°F (90°C).

2 Place the egg whites in a large mixing bowl and add the cream of tartar. Using a hand mixer on medium speed, whip the egg whites for around 3 minutes, until stiff peaks form. Gradually add ½ cup of the sugar while continuing to beat the mixture.

3 Cover a baking sheet with parchment paper. Divide the mixture into 4 circles on the baking sheet. Use a spatula to create a divot in the middle of each circle.

4 Bake the pavlovas for 45 minutes. Then turn off the oven but don't open it for another hour.

5 While the pavlovas are baking, combine the raspberries, water, the remaining 1 tablespoon of sugar, and the orange zest in a small saucepan.

6 Over medium heat, bring the raspberry sauce to a simmer while continuing to stir. Boil the mixture for 1 minute; then remove from heat. If desired, puree with an immersion blender when slightly cooled.

7 When the pavlovas are ready, arrange each on a plate and drizzle the raspberry sauce over top. Garnish with mint leaves, berries, and whipped cream if desired.

PER SERVING: *Calories 133 (From Fat 2); Fat 0g (Saturated 0g); Cholesterol 0mg; Sodium 28mg; Carbohydrate 32g (Dietary Fiber 2g); Protein 2g.*

Dreamy Banana Cream Dessert

PREP TIME: 10 MIN | COOK TIME: 20 MIN | YIELD: 6 SERVINGS

INGREDIENTS

½ cup (125 mL) rice flour

2 tablespoons (30 mL) coconut flour

2 tablespoons (30 mL) plus ¼ cup (60 mL) medium shredded coconut, unsweetened, divided

1 egg

2 tablespoons (30 mL) melted butter

2 cups (500 mL) lactose-free milk

2 egg yolks

⅔ cup (170 mL) white sugar

2 tablespoons (30 mL) cornstarch

½ teaspoon (2.5 mL) salt

2 teaspoons (10 mL) vanilla extract

2 bananas, peeled and sliced

DIRECTIONS

1 Preheat the oven to 350°F (180°C).

2 In a small bowl, combine the rice flour, coconut flour, 2 tablespoons of the medium shredded coconut, egg, and butter. Mix well.

3 Press the mixture into a 9-x-9-inch pan and bake for 20 minutes, or until the edges of the crust start to brown.

4 While the crust is baking, combine the milk and egg yolks in a medium saucepan and stir to combine.

5 To the saucepan, add the sugar, cornstarch, and salt. Turn the heat to medium-high and whisk constantly for around 8 minutes, until the mixture starts to boil.

6 Boil the mixture for 1 minute; then remove from the heat. Add the vanilla and mix. Allow the mixture to cool.

7 Remove the crust from the oven when done. When cool to the touch, lay the banana pieces in an even layer over top. Spread the pudding mixture on top of the bananas. Sprinkle the remaining ¼ cup of coconut on top of the dessert.

8 Refrigerate for at least 1 hour. Then spoon into bowls and serve.

PER SERVING: *Calories 398 (From Fat 171); Fat 19g (Saturated 14g); Cholesterol 127mg; Sodium 283mg; Carbohydrate 53g (Dietary Fiber 5g); Protein 7g.*

Caramelized Bananas

INGREDIENTS

6 pecan halves, finely chopped

1 teaspoon (5 mL) coconut oil

2 tablespoons (30 mL) brown sugar

1 tablespoon (15 mL) water

1 banana, peeled and cut lengthwise

One square (10 g) dark chocolate, finely chopped

Coconut-based whipped cream for garnish (optional)

DIRECTIONS

1 In a small frying pan over medium-high heat, toast the chopped pecans for about 1 minute until slightly fragrant. Set aside to cool.

2 In another frying pan over medium heat, add the coconut oil and brown sugar; stir until the coconut oil melts.

3 Add the water to the pan and then place the banana halves face down. Cook for 3 to 4 minutes while basting the banana in the sauce; then flip and cook for another 3 to 4 minutes, until golden brown.

4 Remove from the heat. Place each banana half on a plate, drizzle with the remaining liquid in the pan, and sprinkle with the pecans and chocolate. If desired, top with whipped cream. Serve immediately.

PER SERVING: *Calories 178 (From Fat 77); Fat 9g (Saturated 4g); Cholesterol 0mg; Sodium 5mg; Carbohydrate 26g (Dietary Fiber 3g); Protein 2g.*

Piña Colada Popsicles

PREP TIME: 5 MIN | FREEZE TIME: 3 HR | YIELD: 4 SERVINGS

INGREDIENTS

1 cup (250 mL) plain coconut-based yogurt

½ cup (125 mL) canned crushed pineapple, drained

½ teaspoon (2.5 mL) coconut extract

2 tablespoons (30 mL) white sugar

DIRECTIONS

1 In a blender (or a medium bowl if using an immersion blender), mix all the ingredients.

2 Using the blender or immersion blender on medium speed, blend the ingredients until smooth, about 30 seconds.

3 Pour the mixture into popsicle molds and add the sticks.

4 Freeze at least 3 hours or until firm.

PER SERVING: *Calories 102 (From Fat 41); Fat 5g (Saturated 4g); Cholesterol 0mg; Sodium 2mg; Carbohydrate 14g (Dietary Fiber 3g); Protein 0g.*

TIP: Popsicle molds vary in size and design, and the number of popsicles you'll get from this recipe depends on the size of the molds you have on hand. You may want to double the recipe if you're working with larger molds.

6

The Part of Tens

Discover the top ten recommended items for surviving and thriving with IBS.

Correct common misunderstandings about IBS.

Chapter **22**

Ten Items for Your IBS Survival Kit

I n 2024, the *Taipei Times* featured a news article about a man who allegedly committed a somewhat unusual crime. The accused was a 21-year-old university student who one day rushed into a convenience store, grabbed a small packet of tissues without paying, and ran to the washroom. The store clerk reported the situation to police, and the young man was charged with theft. The store's video surveillance footage was subsequently used as evidence against him. But in court, the judge learned that the accused had irritable bowel syndrome (IBS) and sometimes had the unexpected need for a bowel movement, requiring the urgent use of a toilet. The judge, showing compassion, issued an acquittal for the man based on his medical condition and the minor nature of the offense.

Many people with IBS know that emergencies happen — and these situations have the potential to be somewhat messy and embarrassing. But you don't need to risk trouble with the law by grabbing what you need from a store shelf. Instead, you can help prevent emergencies by equipping yourself with some key items that help you succeed throughout your day. Just as a mountain expedition tour guide wouldn't set out on a day's work without all the survival necessities, an individual with IBS should always keep some trusty supplies at hand.

In this chapter, you find the makings of an IBS survival kit — the top ten items that may help you keep your symptoms under control as you go about your day.

Not all the items in the list apply to everyone, so feel free to use this list as a starting place and personalize it to your unique situation.

Wet Wipes

Sometimes having IBS is a messy business. (If you know, you know.) Wet wipes are better for cleaning messes than toilet paper, so be sure to keep some on hand at all times.

TIP

You may be able to buy a travel-size package of premoistened skin wipes to carry around with you. But if you have to buy a large package, transfer a few of them to a small resealable plastic bag to carry with you on the go. Make sure to dispose of them correctly (so you don't have the extra embarrassment of a clogged toilet). Avoid wipes with antimicrobial substances — they can do more harm than good for both personal and community health.

Before-You-Go Toilet Spray

The experience is common, whether or not you have IBS: You're in a busy restaurant or other public place with a single-person washroom, which has a lineup of people waiting to use it. You go in and take your turn. Afterward, you awkwardly slink out without making eye contact with the person next in line, knowing you've left behind a telltale smell that they probably won't appreciate. Especially when you have IBS, a smelly bathroom can seem like a loud announcement about the type of symptoms you're dealing with.

This situation can be prevented most of the time with another item in the IBS survival kit: before-you-go toilet spray. Before-you-go toilet sprays usually contain a blend of essential oils and odor-neutralizing compounds. This type of spray is designed to be applied to the toilet bowl water before you sit down, creating a thin film on the surface that traps and neutralizes odors before they can spread. When you flush, the water carries away the odors trapped beneath the surface, leaving behind only the subtly pleasant fragrance of the essential oils. This type of spray differs from a typical air freshener, which only masks toilet-related odors with fragrant chemicals after they've been distributed throughout the bathroom by the act of flushing.

The pleasant scent of a before-you-go spray usually contributes to its effectiveness, but if you're scent sensitive, Flushie offers an unscented spray.

Water Bottle

Hydration is incredibly important in IBS because it's necessary for smooth diges-tion, whether in IBS-D (diarrhea) or IBS-C (constipation), and for the general functioning of your body. So, the next recommended item for your IBS survival kit is a portable and durable water bottle.

TIP

Vessels for holding water are available in many different styles and options, so you may need to try a few before finding one that's most convenient for you. Try to avoid a built-in straw — it can make you consume more air, leading to worse symptoms. Also, choose a water bottle that's easy to carry with you most of the time so you'll be able to sip water throughout the day. Typically, a tightly sealed lid of some kind makes sense so it's less likely to spill in a purse or backpack.

REMEMBER

Don't forget to clean your water bottle at the end of the day, and let it dry out completely before filling it up again.

Handy Snacks

People with IBS typically avoid eating things they know will cause their symptoms to flare up. But what if there's nothing else to eat at that moment? When you're hungry, you may feel anxious, snap at other people, act impulsively, or make careless mistakes. Plus, food avoidance may backfire — your symptoms may bother you anyway if you go for long periods of time without eating.

You can prevent the consequences of being hungry (hangry, even) by always car-rying a supply of snacks you can safely eat. Choose some portable snacks that are easy on your belly, and stash a few of them in a bag or purse that you tend to take with you on outings. Or to be on the safe side, squirrel away some snacks in places you frequent outside of your home, such as your car or your office desk drawer. You can buy some snacks in individual portions, or re-portion them yourself at home using small resealable bags or containers.

TIP

What type of snacks are appropriate? Avoid candy and very sweet foods that will leave you feeling unsatisfied. Choose nutritious foods you can eat that are shelf-stable — bonus points for snacks that are higher in protein, because they may curb your hunger more effectively. Here are some examples of shelf-stable, IBS-friendly snacks that may work for you:

>> Homemade trail mix with almonds (in small amounts), peanuts, walnuts, pumpkin seeds, and dried cranberries (unsweetened)

» An individual portion of peanut butter with rice crackers or rice cakes

» A small portion (no more than ⅓ cup) of shelled walnuts

» Air-popped popcorn

» A low-FODMAP granola bar

FODMAP stands for *fermentable oligosaccharides, disaccharides, monosaccharides and polyols.* Read more about a low-FODMAP diet in Chapter 8.

Along with your snack stash, keep a supply of the necessary utensils and napkins. Hand sanitizer may also be useful if you're eating in an environment where it's not easy to wash your hands first. Finally, watch the expiration dates of your snacks, and replace them with updated items when necessary.

TIP

Comfortable Clothing

No pants button in the world is a match for bloating and *distension* (the visible expansion of the belly) in IBS. A distended belly will continue to push against its tormentor and complain until the button is finally undone. In IBS, distension is a very common symptom and is sometimes triggered by what you eat, or it can gradually creep up during the course of a normal day.

When you have IBS, it's best if you have clothing that's as flexible as you need it to be. Jeans with a button or another unforgiving fastener may just make you miserable. By giving your belly some room to extend and be comfortable, you may find you're less anxious and less focused on your symptoms.

Here are some tips for keeping your clothing comfortable when you have IBS:

TIP

» **Choose looser-fitting clothes, with an elastic waistband if possible.** If you must wear button-up pants, carry a button extender (available cheaply online) that gives you a little more room. In a pinch you can also use a short elastic band: Loop it around the buttonhole on your pants, and then put the end of the loop around the button. (This option works best if you have a shirt or jacket that hides your button from view.)

» **Choose stretchy fabrics.** They'll accommodate a distended belly without creating marks on your skin.

>> **Wear separate tops and bottoms.** Ladies, one-piece tight dresses and pantsuits may look cute, but you may not appreciate having to undo a zipper and wriggle out of them if you need to use the bathroom quickly. A separate top and bottom gives you the ability to adapt to whatever situation comes your way.

TIP

On days when your symptoms are really unpredictable, you may want to keep a change of comfortable clothing (in particular, shorts or leggings) with you in a plastic bag, just in case a quick change is necessary.

Hot Water Bottle or Heating Pad

When abdominal pain strikes, one of the best ways to find quick relief may be to apply gentle heat to your abdomen. You have several options for a heat source: a hot water bottle, an electric heating pad, or a bean- or grain-filled microwavable heating pad. Not only does this technique work to physically soothe the pain, but it also may help your mind feel more calm and relaxed when your symptoms flare up.

You may be able to take your heat source with you away from home, to use at work or while traveling. For example, you can slip a small hot water bottle into your suitcase for when you travel, and fill it up with water from a hotel room kettle.

WARNING

Whatever source of heat you use, take care to avoid irritating or burning your skin with very hot temperatures. It's best to get a fabric cover for your hot water bottle to avoid feeling the high temperature directly on your skin. With microwavable bean bags, carefully follow the instructions for heating them and shake before using to avoid pockets of accumulated heat. And if you have an electric heating pad, read up on its safety features and try not to fall asleep with the heating pad switched on.

All Things Peppermint

When you have IBS, you may want to have at hand a low-risk treatment with the potential to work quickly to quell unexpected symptoms. Peppermint may fill the bill — it's an herb that's been tested scientifically and shown to help relieve IBS symptoms by relaxing the smooth muscles of the digestive tract.

Peppermint oil capsules are a proven treatment for IBS and may be worth carrying. But even if the capsules don't work for you, other peppermint-based products may bring relief. Peppermint tea may be an easy and gentle way to calm your symptoms, and it's widely available in stores and cafes. Some people with IBS even find that peppermint candies are helpful (although you should take care to brush your teeth after eating sugary candies). Avoid peppermint gum and breath mints, however, because the artificial sweeteners they contain, such as sorbitol, can irritate the gut in IBS. Plus, avoid chewing peppermint gum because it can cause you to swallow more air, creating digestive discomfort.

One other useful item may be peppermint essential oil — not to consume, but to apply to your abdomen as you give yourself a gentle self-massage. Combine one drop of peppermint oil with three to four drops of a carrier oil (such as coconut oil, shea butter, olive oil, or almond oil) and massage it into your abdominal area to help relieve constipation, intestinal gas, or other symptoms.

WARNING

If you're taking peppermint oil capsules, make sure to stick to the recommended dose as indicated on the label. If you consume too many capsules, the product may paradoxically cause the same symptoms you're trying to avoid. Large amounts may also cause heartburn.

In addition to peppermint, you may also want to carry a supply of any over-the-counter medications that you've found effective for treating your symptoms quickly.

A Go-To Breathing Exercise

IBS isn't just about the gut — it's about the brain, too. Calm breathing is an excellent way to train your body and your brain into balance, helping reduce the impact of your symptoms.

Everyone with IBS needs at least one go-to breathing exercise that can serve as a quick and discreet way to induce a more relaxed state. Even if you have a regular meditation and breathing practice, you can pick one quick breathing exercise that helps calm you when you start to feel your symptoms coming on. Here are some examples of suitable breathing exercises:

>> **Belly breathing:** Take five long, slow breaths in and out. Each time you breathe in, allow your belly (not your chest) to rise gently. When you breathe out, tighten your belly slightly. You may want to place one hand on your belly to feel its movement as you breathe in and out.

>> **Box breathing (or square breathing):** To implement this simple yet powerful technique, take slow, deep breaths in a structured pattern in four equal parts:

1. **Inhale.** Breathe in deeply through the nose for a count of four seconds, extending your belly as you inhale deeply.

2. **Hold.** Hold your breath at the top of the inhale for four seconds.

3. **Exhale.** Slowly exhale through the mouth for four seconds.

4. **Hold.** Hold your breath at the bottom of the exhale for four seconds.

Repeat the pattern for several cycles.

A Yoga Mat

Sometimes your IBS symptoms may make you want to stay curled up on the couch — but nearly always, your digestion will be better off if you regularly practice gentle movement. Yoga, in particular, can help regulate the functioning of your digestive tract, preventing trapped gas and reducing bloating and distension after a meal. Research shows that in addition to reducing symptoms, yoga may also improve the mental health and overall quality of life of people with IBS.

You don't always have to go out and attend a yoga class. Even a few postures done at home can give you many of the benefits of yoga. So, an essential item in your IBS survival kit is a yoga mat you can use at home. Whether you choose an inexpensive mat from the drugstore or a top-of-the-line mat from a specialty yoga store, a yoga mat is a way to help mark out a space on the floor and provide grip while practicing some gentle movement and breathing.

Find a place in your home where it's easy to set up your yoga mat and try to do a few yoga postures at the same time every day. Try some of the postures you learn in a yoga class, or make use of a book or video. And a little yoga can go a long way: In one study, just 12 yoga postures done twice a day was enough to greatly reduce symptoms in people with IBS. Other studies have shown that different yoga schedules provide benefits, too. (Chapter 11 has more details on yoga for IBS.)

A Diary

When you're having a bad day with IBS, the symptoms can be all-consuming, and it can be hard to remember that you've ever had a single good day.

An IBS diary is another important item for your IBS survival kit because it allows you to document both the good days and the bad ones, allowing you to have a broader perspective on your IBS and perhaps gain some insights into what works to reduce your symptoms.

Your IBS diary can be on paper or digital — but getting into the habit of jotting down a few notes on a daily basis is important. You don't have to write down your deepest secrets, but some observations you may want to write down are:

>> A simple description of your symptoms that day

>> How you felt physically

>> Whether you ate anything unusual

>> Your state of mind and whether you experienced any significant moments of stress

Chapter **23**

Ten Myths about IBS

No longer a secret that's kept behind the bathroom door, irritable bowel syndrome (IBS) is a topic that now seems to pop up everywhere. From news articles to Instagram to online chat groups, talking about IBS has never been more popular. (If you're inclined, you can even buy a variety of IBS merchandise, such as a mug that says "IBS Queen" in bubblegum pink lettering.) Then again, for something that affects around 10 percent of the population, maybe its emergence into the mainstream was inevitable. But one side effect of IBS's recent popularity is the increase in false and misleading information about the condition.

Whether it's an influencer on social media exhorting you not to accept the diagnosis of IBS because it's really just a food intolerance, or a healthcare professional who says you'd be fine if you could only manage to relax a bit, IBS myths can come from many different places and take many different forms. Some misinformation, such as the miraculous powers of a certain herb, may also be commercially motivated. Myths can be harmful because they can

» Cause misunderstandings or conflict with core members of your healthcare team

» Leave you confused about what treatments to commit to

» Give you false hope in an unproven treatment that may give you disappointing results

>> Cost a lot, with questionable benefit

>> Make you give up hope of finding treatments that work for you, leading to unnecessary suffering

Scientific and clinical understandings of IBS are also changing quickly, so anyone who's not familiar with the latest thinking may be inadvertently spreading outdated information.

The purpose of this chapter is to tackle the misinformation and misunderstandings head on, debunking common myths and empowering you with accurate information. By reading through these ten common misunderstandings and finding out the facts, you'll be more up-to-date on the current scientific information about IBS than the vast majority of people. You'll be able to move forward knowing you have a good basic foundation of knowledge.

So, without further ado, here are ten common myths about IBS and the truth about each one.

IBS Is All in Your Head

The idea that the gastrointestinal (GI) symptoms of IBS originate from worry, stress, or a psychiatric disorder is a longstanding myth that probably stems from the fact that the GI tract in someone with IBS looks physically normal. And it's true that traditional medical tests can't detect any physical anomaly in the digestive system. But the coordination of digestion definitely goes awry in IBS, and the reported symptoms of pain and altered bowel movements in a particular pattern are enough to diagnose the condition (in conjunction with certain medical tests to rule out other conditions that can look similar to IBS).

REMEMBER

In recent years, medical professionals and researchers have come to characterize IBS as a disorder of gut-brain interaction (DGBI), acknowledging it as a distinct disorder that manifests both physically and mentally. The physical symptoms are the basis of the diagnosis, but IBS has effects on mental wellness, too — whether it's a vicious circle of increased stress and worry about digestion, or clinically diagnosed anxiety or depression (see Chapters 2 and 4). So, even though IBS doesn't exclusively originate from stress or any other brain-related experience, IBS itself creates a cycle of stress and GI symptoms that's difficult to break without several types of simultaneous treatment that address the body and mind holistically.

A clarification is warranted, though: After you have the very real diagnosis of IBS, your brain does have a role in how symptoms manifest. The disordered gut-brain communication works in both directions, so just as the gut symptoms can cause worry, mental stress can contribute to altered motility and secretion of hormones that result in gut symptoms. In other words, stress can indeed trigger symptoms in a situation of disordered gut-brain communication.

So, no, IBS is not all in your head. But yes, your head has a part to play in the symptoms you experience. Ultimately, IBS is probably caused by complex interactions between your biology and your lifestyle, including your healthy habits and the way that events of your childhood may have helped wire your brain networks, as well as alterations in your gut microbiome. Fortunately, no matter how IBS originates, scientists know a fair amount now about the treatments that work to help get symptoms under control.

Nothing's Wrong If All the Tests Come Back Normal

When seeking a diagnosis, miscommunication commonly occurs between individuals with GI symptoms and their healthcare professionals. Your doctor may not make it clear that the diagnosis of IBS is primarily made based on the pattern of symptoms you report, and the diagnosis is confirmed after reviewing your medical history as well as relevant medical test results. You may feel that your reported symptoms are dismissed in the process of diagnosis, but your doctor has likely noted the symptoms and is, in fact, using them as the basis of the diagnosis.

REMEMBER

After symptoms are noted, depending on your individual medical situation, several tests are usually required to confirm a diagnosis of IBS. But instead of these tests positively confirming IBS, they rule out other conditions (such as celiac disease or colorectal cancer) that commonly look like IBS. For someone with IBS, these tests are expected to come back within the normal range, and they're a necessary step in the process of diagnosis. Turn to Chapter 5 for more on diagnosing IBS.

IBS Diarrhea Is the Same as Infectious Diarrhea

Another common myth related to IBS is that the loose, watery stool that occurs in IBS-D (diarrhea) is the same as the diarrhea that occurs when someone has a gut infection.

In a gut infection, the diarrhea is a result of pathogenic microorganisms either releasing toxins or causing inflammation in the GI tract. The diarrhea typically resolves when the immune system stops the proliferation of the harmful microorganisms. However, without proper hygiene, the infectious bacteria can be passed on to another person.

By contrast, diarrhea in IBS can't be passed on to anyone else, nor does it result from excessive toxins or inflammation. It doesn't cause major complications such as poor kidney function. (However, any large volume of diarrhea can lead to dehydration or abnormal electrolytes if not treated.)

IBS-D may be caused by many overlapping factors, such as abnormal muscle contractions in the GI tract or fast transit of intestinal contents through the intestines (leaving little time for water to be absorbed in the colon). In IBS, your small intestine is normally absorbing your food properly despite the loose stools, which is why IBS is not usually associated with weight loss. (If you're unintentionally losing weight with IBS, tell your doctor.)

To complicate the picture, however, sometimes infectious diarrhea can lead to IBS (which is called *post-infectious IBS*). In such cases, it can be hard to draw the line between the infectious diarrhea and IBS-related diarrhea. (See Chapter 3 for more details.)

IBS Can Be Cured

IBS is not the same as an occasionally upset stomach, which can pop up sometimes depending on what's happening in your life. Gut symptoms such as occasional constipation or abdominal pain are very prevalent in the general population, but what sets IBS apart is the pattern of these symptoms and the fact that they recur constantly over a lifetime. IBS is a lifelong, chronic disorder that can't be cured and will rear its head again and again if it isn't managed.

REMEMBER

The chronic nature of IBS doesn't necessarily mean you'll be dealing with symptoms every single day of your life, however. You may go through occasional periods of IBS remission when your symptoms don't bother you. And you may be able to get your symptoms under control by implementing a personalized combination of dietary changes, lifestyle modifications, mind-body treatments, and possibly medications. Through trial and error, you may eventually find out how to leverage all these things to live symptom-free. Persistence is required to figure out the exact combination that works for you, but healthcare professionals can guide you along — and having a couple of supportive family members or friends can make a big difference, too.

IBS Is the Same as IBD

Given the similar acronyms, IBS and IBD (inflammatory bowel disease) are often confused with each other. But even for people who understand that the letter *I* stands for *irritable* in one case and *inflammatory* in the other, the two conditions may be tricky to differentiate.

REMEMBER

IBS and IBD are two very different kinds of conditions that affect the digestive tract. IBD is an umbrella term for specific diseases — namely, Crohn's disease and ulcerative colitis — in which sections of inflammation and tissue damage in the GI tract are detected when a gastroenterologist performs imaging or a colonoscopy. IBS, on the other hand, is characterized by a GI tract that looks normal when examined under a microscope, accompanied by a distinct pattern of symptoms. IBD may manifest with blood in the stool and elevation of inflammatory markers such as calprotectin, which aren't observed in IBS. Untreated or severe IBD may be associated with complications, such as surgery and colorectal cancer, which are not associated with IBS. Nor does IBS turn into IBD — they're two distinct and unrelated patterns of disease. However, IBS and IBD are sometimes difficult to tell apart based on symptoms alone, so one can be mistaken for the other.

For both IBS and IBD, however, lifestyle changes are an important part of the treatment strategy.

One Treatment Fits All

"My daughter has IBS, and she has no symptoms now that she cut out wheat."

"My friend with IBS says alkaline water made all the difference."

Strangers and friends alike often make comments like these when they find out you have IBS. But unfortunately, personal anecdotes about what worked well for one person with IBS likely have limited applicability to your own situation. First, you don't learn the entire context when you hear such stories. Maybe the same week that the daughter cut out wheat from her diet, she simultaneously quit her stressful job. Or maybe the friend was drinking four gut-irritating diet colas per day before he replaced them with alkaline water. Plus, even when all else is equal, a treatment that works like a charm for one person with IBS may have no benefits for another person. As we note in Chapter 2, the underlying cause of IBS is often different from one person to the next.

That's not to say the treatments that work are completely random. Some treatments have been tested in scientific studies across populations of people with IBS and shown to work when other factors are held constant. Evidence supports a multi-treatment strategy that involves diet adjustments, mind-body treatments with stress reduction, lifestyle modifications, and judicious use of medications.

Ultimately, if you wrote the story of your ideal IBS treatment, it would be different from everyone else's story. Embrace your unique story — and with guidance from your support team, you can find the treatments that really work for you.

IBS Is Just Another Name for Food Intolerance

It's a relatively common story: Someone is diagnosed with IBS and tries cutting out certain foods from their diet to get their symptoms under control. They cut out all dairy products and wheat, for example, and — *voilà!* — their symptoms seem to completely disappear.

Such cases may lead to the assumption that IBS is really just a food intolerance, and by figuring out which foods irritate your gut, you can get your symptoms 100 percent under control. This mistaken assumption sometimes leads people to restrict their diet more and more, attempting to remove all possible food triggers, until they're eating only a small number of foods that they think they can tolerate. But sometimes those few foods, or even a sip of water, bring on their symptoms. If everything including water seems to irritate your gut, then clearly there's more going on than food intolerance.

REMEMBER

In reality, IBS can't be managed completely through food choices. For a tiny fraction of people with IBS, symptom control through diet may be maintained over the long term — but the symptoms come back for the vast majority of people no matter how much dietary control they exert. The dietary change, in other words, may help the gut perform better, but the underlying issues with function are long-lasting and can be triggered by stress or other changes in your life. And conversely, if you're in a good place and maintaining healthy habits, sometimes you can tolerate the foods you thought would trigger your symptoms.

Everyone with IBS Can Benefit from Eating More Fiber

Fiber is associated with multiple health benefits over a lifetime. Traditionally, one of the most prevalent pieces of advice for people with IBS was to increase intake of fiber — especially soluble fiber (a type that dissolves in water to form a gel that adds bulk to the stool and slows digestion). But registered dietitians came to realize that this advice caused absolute misery for some people with IBS and ended up increasing their symptoms.

As it turns out, fiber tolerance in IBS is highly personal. Each person with IBS may respond to different fiber types and different daily amounts. Because soluble fibers have shown the best results for improving symptoms, doctors often currently start with the advice to increase soluble fiber, but they also add that the intake should be discontinued if symptoms appear worse. After adjusting fiber intake to get symptoms under control, specific types of fiber can gradually be added back into the diet to meet the minimum recommended daily intakes of 25 grams for females and 38 grams for males.

Discomfort Is Inevitable When You Have IBS

Sometimes when a person with IBS is having a particularly bad day, they may post a pessimistic comment like this in an IBS online chat group: "It's like I'm chained to the toilet. I guess I just have to live this way."

The truth is, you don't have to fall into the trap of thinking you'll live with discomfort for the rest of your life. It's totally possible to have an enjoyable, vibrant life with IBS.

IBS is not an easy disorder to treat. But at the same time, the science is advancing very quickly. Symptoms can improve or be controlled using methods that are proven to work all around the world. The mistake that many people make is focusing too narrowly on gut-centric treatments. Diet, medications, and dietary supplements that target the gut can take you part of the way, but most people also need brain-focused therapies (mind-body treatments, as described in Chapter 11), as well as other lifestyle changes to really get symptoms under control.

Some clinics specialize in treating IBS and have all the relevant professionals and latest tools at hand, helping people implement tailored treatment plans. These centers report patient satisfaction rates of around 80 percent to 85 percent — powerful proof that discomfort doesn't have to be part and parcel of IBS.

You Don't Need to Take IBS Seriously

IBS is a genuine medical condition. Even though IBS doesn't shorten your life or lead to medical complications such as surgery or colorectal cancer, it's still something you should take seriously and try to treat. Studies show that IBS has an impact on quality of life, causing people to feel it's holding them back from living the life they want to live. This can be true regardless of whether the symptoms are mild or intense.

So, anyone who receives a diagnosis of IBS and tries to brush it off without changing anything may soon find that, unless hanging out near the toilet is among your life goals, it's better to take IBS seriously and figure out a treatment plan.

Index

parasympathetic nervous system, 16, 54, 162, 165

Parmesan Quinoa Patties, 278, 279

Pavlovas with Raspberry Sauce, 298, 300

Peanut Sauce, Chicken and Broccoli in Creamy, 272, 276

Peanut-Lime Dressing, Soba Salad with, 256, 259

pediatric IBS. *See* childhood IBS

PEG (polyethylene glycol) 3350 laxative, 141–142, 146

pelvic floor dysfunction, 9, 43–44

pelvic floor dyssynergia, 184

pelvic floor therapy, 184, 185

pelvic organ prolapse, 184

peppermint, 146, 311–312

peristalsis, 51, 183

permeability, intestinal, 9, 43, 53

personalization phase, low-FODMAP diet, 130–131

pesticide exposure, 40

Pesto Rice, Shrimp, Pepper, and Pineapple Skewers with, 264, 267–268

PFC (prefrontal cortex), 61

physical activity. *See* exercise

physicians, in support team, 91–92

physiotherapy, 185

pineapple

Piña Colada Popsicles, 298, 303

Shrimp, Pepper, and Pineapple Skewers with Pesto Rice, 264, 267–268

Sweet-and-Sour Pineapple Fish, 264, 271

placebo effect, 160

Polenta Rounds, Herb and Tomato, 283, 287

polyethylene glycol (PEG) 3350 laxative, 141–142, 146

polyols, 125, 129

polyphenols, 110

Pork and Cabbage Rice-Paper Wraps, 272, 273

portion sizes, 112, 126, 131, 198

positivity, 88–90, 160, 186

postbiotics, 156

post-infectious IBS, 41, 208, 318

post-meal walks, 179

postpartum period, navigating IBS during, 224–225

Potato Bacon Salad, 256, 257

prebiotics, 124, 125, 135, 136, 155–156

preconception planning, 216–217

prefrontal cortex (PFC), 61

pregnancy, IBS during

adjusting lifestyle habits, 220–221

birth and postpartum period, 224–225

cautions warranted in, 218

danger signs, 218

diet, optimizing, 221–223

hydration, 218, 223

overview, 17–18, 215–216

planning for pregnancy, 216–217

symptom changes in, 218–219

premature dietary changes, avoiding, 83

prepared foods, low-FODMAP, 241–242

prescription medications, 147–150

presenteeism, 34

pre-sport meals, 232–233

prevalence of IBS, 38–39

prevention of IBS, 44–45

primary care physicians, 91–92

probiotics, 146–147, 155, 211

promotility agents (prokinetics), 149

protein, 109, 127, 131, 284

psychological conditions co-occurring with IBS, 31–33

psychological risk factors for childhood IBS, 208

psychologists, 94, 164, 193

public places, quality of life in, 196

Pumpkin Spice Oatmeal Muffins, 292, 297

Q

quality of life (QoL)

dating and intimacy, 199–200

defined, 191

eating out, 198

effect of IBS on, 33–35

future, grappling with, 200–201

at home, 193–194

in others' homes, 196–198

overview, 17, 189–190, 193

in public places, 196

at school, 195

tools and services for IBS, 190–193

traveling, 198–199

at work, 194–195

Quinoa Patties, Parmesan, 278, 279

R

Raman, Maitreyi, 231

Raspberry Sauce, Pavlovas with, 298, 300

ready-made low-FODMAP foods, 241–242

recipe blogs, low-FODMAP, 243

recipes, sticking to when changing diet, 247

rectum, 50, 53, 54

refined grains, 109

registered dietitians, 92–93, 238–239, 246

regurgitation, 205

reintroduction phase, low-FODMAP diet, 128–129

Remember icon, explained, 3

remission of IBS symptoms, 24–25, 318–319

resistant starches, 123

About the Authors

Kristina Campbell, MSc: Kristina Campbell, a science writer from Victoria, Canada, has spent the past 12 years covering gut health and microbiome science for media throughout Europe and North America. In addition to having written hundreds of articles, she is the author of a previous *For Dummies* book, *Gut Health For Dummies* (John Wiley & Sons). Her other books are *The Well-Fed Microbiome Cookbook* (Rockridge Press) and the first and second editions of the textbook *Gut Microbiota: Interactive Effects on Nutrition and Health* (Academic Press), cowritten with Drs. Edward Ishiguro and Natasha Haskey. Kristina holds degrees from the University of Toronto and the University of British Columbia.

Kristina is passionate about making science relevant and accessible for everyone and supporting scientific and health literacy. You can find her on social media at @bykriscampbell and on Mastodon at @bykriscampbell@sciencemastodon.com.

Natasha Haskey, RD, PhD: Natasha Haskey is a research associate at the University of British Columbia – Okanagan in Canada. She brings over two decades of clinical dietetics experience to her work. Specializing in gastrointestinal issues, she actively engages with patients seeking solutions in this area. Through her research program, she collaborates with a multidisciplinary team to develop innovative treatment approaches that leverage microbiome science and nutrition. Committed to advancing scientific knowledge, Natasha strives to establish strong evidence-based dietary recommendations for individuals with gastrointestinal disorders.

Maitreyi Raman, MD, FRCPC: Maitreyi Raman is a gastroenterologist, physician nutrition specialist, and associate professor of medicine at the University of Calgary in Canada. Her research program is centered on the discovery of diet, nutrient, and gut-brain-microbiome interactions in health and disease. She has published more than 100 peer-reviewed scientific articles, in addition to five books covering topics of diet, nutrition, and how they affect the prevention and treatment of various gastrointestinal conditions for patients and their families. She has also published several scientific book chapters, and has codeveloped a digital platform, LyfeMD (www.lyfemd.com) to empower and support people with digestive disease with evidence-based and state-of-the-art lifestyle solutions. Dr. Raman has been the recipient of several local, national, and international awards for teaching and research. Clinically, Dr. Raman has implemented a specialized clinic for the assessment and management of malnutrition and nutritional disorders for patients with gastrointestinal conditions, which has served as a foundation for two other programs in North America. She is also a certified Yoga Nidra instructor and recommends mind-body solutions to complement medical care.

Dedication

From Kristina: Many years ago, when I was suffering from debilitating gut symptoms without an IBS diagnosis and not knowing where to turn for help, I decided to share my experiences with a few people around me. I found that I was far from alone in dealing with digestive problems and that I could learn a lot from others who had similar symptoms. This book is dedicated to family and friends with IBS or digestive symptoms who've let me in on their experiences and stories over the years, including Deanna, Kim, Sarah, Anusha, and Sara, to name just a few. Thank you for illuminating the way for everyone who walks this path after you.

From Maitreyi: To my parents and husband who have inspired and supported the path of mind-body and holistic medicine. Through the wisdom of my family, and with the benefit of listening to my thousands of patients over 20 years, I now understand how medical sciences need to prioritize holistic research, and integrate holistic strategies into clinical care urgently to support conventional medical approaches.

From Natasha: To my husband, Ryan, whose unwavering support, encouragement, and patience have made this journey possible — thank you for keeping me well fed, lifting me up during challenges, and always believing in my passion.

Authors' Acknowledgments

From Kristina: I'm grateful to Callum, Clara, and Lewis for helping me welcome book number five into our family. Thank you to my wonderful agent, Matt Wagner, who set in motion my two-book *For Dummies* journey, and whose guidance keeps me on the right track. Kudos to Wiley for revisiting this important condition that affects so many people. Thanks in particular to Elizabeth Stilwell for offering me the project and being a great support throughout the process. Thanks also to our editor, Elizabeth Kuball, for the valuable advice and assistance that made this manuscript shine.

Sending out appreciation to Deanna Picklyk for valuable resources and editing for Chapter 6, and to Ayva Lewis, Ernestine Chablis, Mayu Patton, and Raylene Van den Adel for recipe inspiration.

From Natasha: I am deeply grateful to my colleagues, mentors, and collaborators for their invaluable guidance and support. I feel truly fortunate to have such an incredible group of cheerleaders by my side. Finally, I extend my heartfelt appreciation to the patients and participants whose willingness to share their experiences has been instrumental in shaping this work.

Publisher's Acknowledgments

Associate Editor: Elizabeth Stilwell

Managing Editor: Kristie Pyles

Editor: Elizabeth Kuball

Technical Editor: Rachel Nix, RD

Production Editor: Tamilmani Varadharaj

Recipe Tester: Rachel Nix, RD

Nutrition Analysis: Rachel Nix, RD

Cover Image: © Svetlana Shamshurina/ Getty Images